# Regenerative Medicine in Pain Practice

Ripu D. Arora
Editor

# Regenerative Medicine in Pain Practice

Springer

*Editor*
Ripu D. Arora
Arora Pain Clinic
Torrance, CA, USA

ISBN 978-3-032-22643-3    ISBN 978-3-032-22644-0 (eBook)
https://doi.org/10.1007/978-3-032-22644-0



This Springer imprint is published by the registered company Springer Nature Switzerland AG
The registered company address is: Gewerbestrasse 11, 6330 Cham, Switzerland

*Dedicated to my dearest wife Sheila, my parents, my family, my mentors, my patients, and my teachers.*

# Foreword

*Regenerative Medicine in Pain Practice* by Ripu D. Arora, MD, offers a comprehensive knowledge-based handbook presented in a manner that leaves the reader eager to learn more. While many books address regenerative medicine, this volume is among the rare few that focus specifically on its role in pain practice. The presentation is clear, the writing is easy to follow, and the content provides practical insights and answers to questions commonly raised by clinicians. With its 12 chapters, numerous figures, and extensive reading list, the book serves as both a guide and a resource.

In the second edition of *Essentials of Regenerative Medicine in Interventional Pain Management*, Manchikanti et al. described regenerative medicine as an "emerging specialty." Dr. Arora and his coauthors advance this concept further, arguing that the field has moved beyond its emerging stage and has reached a level of maturity. Regenerative medicine spans a broad spectrum of scientific disciplines, including engineering, molecular sciences, biologics, and healthcare-related research, all of which are addressed in this work.

What sets regenerative medicine apart is its focus on repairing, replacing, or restoring damaged or diseased tissues and organs, in contrast to most medical and surgical interventions that primarily manage symptoms. As detailed in this book, regenerative therapies encompass a wide variety of techniques, including stem cell therapy, platelet-rich plasma (PRP) and its derivatives, tissue engineering, and gene therapy. These modalities are clearly explained and thoughtfully applied to both spinal and non-spinal disorders, including neurodegenerative diseases.

As this book illustrates, regenerative medicine is a rapidly advancing field with active global research and development. Scientists continue to refine the safety and effectiveness of these therapies while exploring new applications. Yet, important challenges remain—ethical considerations, potential unintended consequences, and questions of accessibility and affordability, particularly within the United States.

In conclusion, regenerative medicine offers tremendous promise for patients suffering from pain, with the potential to transform treatment by addressing underlying pathology rather than simply managing symptoms. However, it is essential to recognize that these therapies are still evolving, may not be suitable for every patient, and may not be widely affordable at present.

Dr. Arora is to be commended for his valuable contribution to the field. His clear writing style, practical approach, and use of illustrative figures make this book an important addition to the literature and a useful resource for clinicians and trainees alike.

Laxmaiah Manchikanti

Chairman of the Board and Chief Executive Officer, ASIPP and SIPMS, Director, Pain Management Centers of America
Ambulatory Surgery Center and Pain Care Surgery Center
Paducah, KY, USA

Clinical Professor, Anesthesiology and Perioperative Medicine
University of Louisville
Louisville, KY, USA

Professor of Anesthesiology-Research, Department of Anesthesiology, School of Medicine
LSU Health Sciences Center
Shreveport, LA, USA

# Foreword

In the past two decades, orthobiologics have transitioned from being experimental adjuncts in musculoskeletal care to becoming one of the most promising pillars of regenerative medicine. For conditions of the spine, joints, and soft tissues—often defined by chronic pain, functional decline, and limited natural healing capacity—orthobiologics offer the possibility of restoring form and function by working with the body's own repair mechanisms.

This book was conceived to bridge a critical gap: the need for a comprehensive, clinically focused resource that integrates the latest scientific evidence with practical insights for the practicing spine, orthopedic, sports medicine, and rehabilitation specialist. While high-quality research in orthobiologics is rapidly emerging, the pace of discovery has often outstripped the availability of organized, clinically digestible guidance. Too often, clinicians must navigate fragmented literature, varying procedural techniques, and evolving regulatory frameworks without a clear roadmap.

The scope of this text extends beyond a simple catalog of biologic agents. It is designed to offer a deep understanding of the biology, rationale, and clinical applications of the most relevant orthobiologics interventions—including platelet-rich plasma (PRP), bone marrow aspirate concentrate (BMAC), adipose-derived cell preparations, extracellular vesicles, and acellular scaffolds. Each chapter aims to blend foundational science with real-world procedural considerations, patient selection strategies, and outcome interpretation. The emphasis on spine, orthopedic, and musculoskeletal tissues reflects both the highest areas of clinical demand and some of the most exciting arenas of innovation. The spine, with its unique structural and vascular challenges, has been at the forefront of both enthusiasm and controversy regarding regenerative solutions. Similarly, degenerative joint disease and chronic tendinopathies remain prevalent causes of disability worldwide, where orthobiologics may shift the paradigm from symptom suppression to biologically driven repair.

This book is also grounded in the principle that orthobiologics cannot be practiced in isolation from the broader context of musculoskeletal medicine. Optimal patient outcomes depend on integrating biologic interventions with mechanical correction, physical rehabilitation, metabolic optimization, and patient education. To that end, each section emphasizes multidisciplinary collaboration and the importance of tailoring therapies to the individual rather than applying one-size-fits-all protocols.

The chapters draw on the collective expertise of clinicians, scientists, and researchers who have been instrumental in advancing the field. Their contributions span randomized controlled trials, registry analyses, translational research, and long-term follow-up studies that inform both safety and efficacy. We also address the regulatory, ethical, and economic considerations that every practitioner must navigate when offering orthobiologics care—because clinical excellence must be matched with compliance and patient trust.

As we stand at the intersection of biology, engineering, and clinical medicine, orthobiologics represent more than a new treatment category; they embody a new way of thinking about tissue repair and functional restoration. This book, being grounded in practicality, equips the physician not only with knowledge, but also with the discernment to apply these tools responsibly, effectively, and innovatively at the point of care.

The journey of orthobiologics is still unfolding. This book invites you to be an active participant in shaping its future—for the benefit of our patients, our profession, and the science of healing itself.

Annu Navani, MD, FIPP, ABIPP, DABRM
Founder and Chief Medical Officer, Le Reve
Chief Medical Officer, Boomerang Healthcare
Founder and CEO, Le Reve
Founder and Chair, World Institute of Regenerative Medicine
President-Elect, American Society of Interventional Pain Physicians
www.annunavani.com
www.lerevewellness.com
https://asipp.org/
www.wirmglobal.org

San Jose, California, USA Annu Navani

# My Regenerative Stem Cell Therapy with Dr. Ripu Arora

## A Patient Perspective and Testimonial

Finding Hope After Years of Pain

For years, chronic knee pain controlled my life. Simple activities like climbing stairs, playing my favorite sport, paddle tennis, even short walks, had become increasingly difficult. After exhausting conventional treatments including physical therapy, anti-inflammatories, and cortisone injections with only temporary relief, I faced knee replacement surgery. That's when I discovered regenerative stem cell therapy and Dr. Ripu Arora.

## Exceptional Care from a Master Physician

Dr. Arora's over three decades of experience in regenerative medicine and interventional pain management was immediately apparent. What set him apart was his ability to explain the complex science in understandable terms while maintaining realistic expectations. His philosophy resonated deeply: "Our goal is to help the patient as a whole, to improve the quality of life and improve their functionality in life."

He didn't oversell the treatment. Instead, he educated me honestly about how regenerative medicine works and carefully assessed whether I was a suitable candidate. His integrity and patient-centered approach gave me complete confidence.

Masterful Execution

The administration procedure showcased Dr. Arora's artful precision. His decades of experience in anesthesiology were evident in every aspect. What could have been intimidating felt seamless and professional. He remained fully present, explaining each step while demonstrating remarkable mastery of this developing science.

The hour-long procedure involved minimal discomfort, testament to his exceptional technical skill. I walked out the same day with comprehensive post-procedure instructions.

Life-Changing Results

Within four to six weeks, the constant aching that had plagued me for years began diminishing. By three months, my progress was remarkable.

Six months later, my life has been transformed. I walk without pain, hike on weekends, and keep up with my grandchildren. The stiffness and inflammation have dramatically decreased, restoring mobility I thought was lost forever.

My Highest Recommendation

Dr. Arora's belief that "regenerative medicine is going to be the art of medicine, which everybody will be utilizing in the years to come" proved prophetic. His forward-thinking approach, ethical practice, strict adherence to compliance, and dedication to patient education made all the difference in my journey.

If you're dealing with chronic knee pain and conventional treatments have failed, I cannot recommend Dr. Ripu Arora highly enough. His mastery of interventional pain management, pioneering work in regenerative medicine, and compassionate guidance provide the ideal combination for relief. He doesn't just treat pain; he partners with patients to restore their quality of life through cutting-edge medical science.

This treatment gave me back my independence and the ability to enjoy life again. For that, and for Dr. Arora's exceptional care, I'm truly thankful.

Cengiz Volkan

A grateful patient

# Preface

## My Journey into Regenerative Medicine

I am a board-certified pain management anesthesiologist with over three decades of experience in treating chronic pain. Recently, I added a certification of Competency in Regenerative medicine through the American Society of Interventional Pain Physicians (ASIPP), marking a formal milestone in my journey. My motivation is driven by personal experience, professional curiosity, and a commitment to offering better healing options to my patients to improve the quality of their lives.

A decade ago, I experienced two major injuries, including a lateral meniscus tear of my right knee and a massive rotator cuff injury in my right shoulder. The latter was deemed inoperable by orthopedic surgeons, leaving me searching for alternatives.

In the process, I discovered the emerging field of regenerative medicine. I underwent regenerative mesenchymal stem cell therapy on both the affected knee and the shoulder. The results were nothing short of transformative. Within 9–12 months, I regained full functionality, returning to the activities I love, such as golfing, skiing, and traveling.

Impressed with my own recovery, I immersed myself in studying and learning more about regenerative medicine. I attended conferences, read emerging literature, and engaged with experts in the field. As I gained confidence and knowledge, I began offering regenerative treatments in my clinical practice of interventional pain management. The outcomes have been very encouraging as many patients have reported substantial improvements with reduced pain, increased functionality, and improved quality of life.

Over the years, I've received countless questions from patients and colleagues alike about the science, the procedures, the evidence, and the potential benefits of regenerative therapies. These conversations inspired me to write this book.

I also decided to use the title "Regenerative Medicine in Pain Practice" because I strongly believe that every pain management physician should understand the immense value that regenerative medicine offers to our practice. It is an important tool and resource to help address the complexity of chronic pain in ways that traditional therapies often cannot.

This guide is created for pain specialists, physicians, residents, and informed patients seeking to understand and apply regenerative medicine in real-world clinical scenarios. It blends evidence-based science with clinical experiences to demystify regenerative medicine and its potential to help in pain management. This book explores how regenerative medicine is reshaping pain practice by focusing on tissue repair and functional restoration rather than mere symptom suppression. Regenerative medicine is not a replacement, but a vital addition to the existing algorithm of pain management options.

I am deeply grateful to my mentors and colleagues who have influenced this journey, including Dr. Laxmaiah Manchikanti, Dr. Annu Navani, Dr. Sudhir Diwan, Dr. Sheldon Jordan, Dr. Devi Nampiaparampil, Dr. Joseph Cabaret, and Dr. Sheri Albers.

My deepest appreciation goes to my wife, Sheila Arora, my partner in life and working physician assistant in my practice, whose support has been unwavering. I thank my friends, families, and children for their encouragement, and my beloved parents, whose values and sacrifices gave me the foundation to serve others.

Thank you for joining me on this journey toward better healing and innovative care.

Torrance, CA, USA Ripu D. Arora

# Disclosure

All figures were prepared by the author as original schematic illustrations using Microsoft PowerPoint for this volume. The images are author-created, copyright-free, and designed solely for educational purposes, without the use of AI tools or stock imagery.

# Contents

# Editors and Contributors

## About the Editor

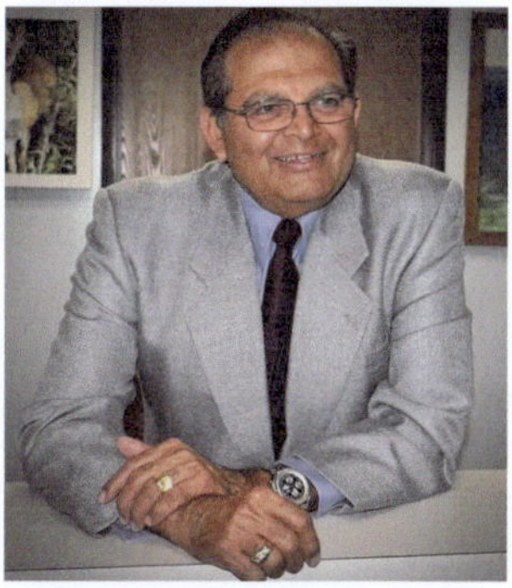

**Ripu D. Arora, MD, MBA** is a board-certified pain management anesthesiologist with Competency certification in Regenerative Medicine by American Society of Interventional Pain Physicians (ASIPP). He has been practicing in Torrance, California, at the Arora Pain Clinic for the past three decades and has an outstanding reputation. He provides passionate care to his patients.

He is a longtime resident of the South Bay area. For over 30 years, he and his wife Sheila Arora, PA-C, have raised their two children there and now enjoy time with their grandchildren.

He specializes in interventional pain management and regenerative medicine. He is known for his keen ability to identify pain triggering mechanisms and for his ability to personalize targeted treatments for optimal patient outcomes. His treatment plans integrate a multidisciplinary approach. He treats his patients based on their own unique physical, psychological, and social needs. His techniques vary from simple nerve injections to advanced interventional pain procedures. He employs regenerative therapy for carefully selected patients.

He earned his medical degree in India, completed orthopedic and surgical training in the UK, and pursued additional training in the United States, including a residency in anesthesiology at Case Western Reserve University, Ohio. He later earned an MBA in Healthcare from the University of California, Irvine, graduating with honors (Beta Gamma Sigma).

He is affiliated with Providence and Torrance Memorial hospitals and has served as Chief of

Anesthesia and Pain Management at Pacifica Community Hospital. He is a member of the Board of Directors for the California Society of Interventional Pain Physicians (CALSIPP) and is a life member of the American Society of Interventional Pain Physicians (ASIPP). He has been Past President of CALSIPP and Past President of his alumni association where he organized educational programs and annual meetings. He is a philanthropist. Currently, he is involved with nonprofit organizations whose goals are to end homelessness in Southern California.

When he is not in the clinic, he enjoys skiing, golfing, scuba diving, flying, photography, and traveling with his family and friends.

**Sheldon Jordan, MD** is a Fellow in the American Academy of Neurology and is board certified in Neurology, Clinical Neurophysiology, Addiction Medicine, and Interventional Pain Management. He is recognized as a top neurologist by Best Doctors in America, Who's Who, Global Edition, and Super Doctors. He trained at both Johns Hopkins and UCLA (University of California at Los Angeles). He has recently retired after 40 years of service at UCLA and the University of Southern California. He is the CEO of The Regenesis Project, Synaptec Network, and Synaptec Research, which are actively involved with cutting-edge research in advanced imaging, focused energy treatments, and regenerative medicine. His work also includes animal and human research on exosomes and stem cells. He and his team work in collaboration with other innovators on research focused on gene therapy using plasmid and viral vectors. He is one of the working visionaries in the development of the GARM clinics whose mission is to provide a range of regenerative treatments to improve the length and quality of life, tailored to a patient's individual needs. He has several clinics in the United States with increasing numbers of clinics scattered throughout the world. He has written over 200 publications and lectures both nationally and internationally. He has been honored with two nominations for the XPRIZE, which is an organization that launches prize-driven global competition, choosing innovators from across the world whose transformational ideas can be tested and will ultimately produce working solutions to global problems. His main areas of interest are in resetting the biological central clock of aging and reversing neurodegenerative diseases.

**Joseph Cabaret** is triple board certified in Anesthesiology, Interventional Pain Management, and in Addiction Medicine. He is the founder and CEO of Genesis Pain Specialists in Camarillo and Anaheim, CA. He is Past President and the current Director of the California Society of Interventional Pain Physicians. He is an instructor in interventional and regenerative medicine techniques for the American Society of Interventional Pain Physicians. He is also a board examiner for the American Board of Interventional Pain Physicians. He has been practicing regenerative medicine since 2012. He has given multiple national lectures and has written several book chapters on regenerative medicine principles and techniques.

**Sheri L. Albers** is a DO, Fellow of the American Society of Interventional Pain Physicians (FASIPP), Fellow of the American Osteopathic College of Radiology (FAOCR), Competency Certification in Regenerative Medicine (ABIPP). She is trained in Radiology (Medical Center of Delaware), Fellowships: Cross-sectional Imaging (MSK/Body, Medical Center of Delaware), Neuroradiology (University of California-Davis), Interventional Pain Medicine (University of California-San Diego). Currently she is Director of Clinical Services and Research for Radiology Research and Consultation. She is board certified in ABIPP, ABR, AOBR. Her Honors and awards include Past President: ASIPP (2022–2023), Board of Directors: ASIPP, Editorial Board and Radiology Section Chief for Pain Physician, AMA CPT Advisory Committee Alternate, Board Examiner: ABIPP, Board of Directors: CALSIPP, Board of Directors: IMCAT.

She has also received Life time achievement award ASIPP, Manchikanti Excellence Award: ASIPP, League of Presidents Award: ASIPP, Distinguished Service Award: ASIPP, Outstanding Achievement Award: ASIPP, Trenery Award for Outstanding Didactic Service for the AOCR, Board of Directors: AOCR, Visiting Professor: Michigan State, Internal Medicine Award for Clinical Excellence, Delta Omega Award, Dean's Commendation, Founding Chairperson and President of the Resident's Section: Philadelphia Roentgen Ray Society, Psi Chi, Phi Beta Kappa, Phi Kappa Phi

## Contributors

**Sheri L. Albers** Radiology Research and Consultation, Sacramento, CA, USA

**Ripu D. Arora** Arora Pain Clinic, Torrance, CA, USA

**Joseph Cabaret** Pain Clinic Camarillo, Camarillo, CA, USA

**Sheldon Jordan** Regenesis Project, Santa Monica, CA, USA

# Introduction to Regenerative Medicine 1

Ripu D. Arora

> Innovation distinguishes between a leader and a follower. —Steve Jobs

The practice of pain management has traditionally relied on physical therapy, acupuncture, pharmaceuticals (including non-steroidal medications and opioids), and interventional and invasive surgical procedures. However, the evolving knowledge of the regenerative process, tissue repair, and advances in regenerative medicine are opening a transformative approach to treatment that harnesses the body's natural healing abilities.

## 1.1 Definition

Regenerative medicine is a groundbreaking branch of medical science. It is

> A science focusing on the use of cellular products to repair and regenerate diseased or damaged cells, tissues, or organs, thereby restoring normal function and healing the body without surgical or pharmaceutical interventions.

## 1.2 Historical Context (Fig. 1.1)

**Ancient Foundations**
*~500* BCE *(2500 years ago)* The journey of regenerative medicine is rooted in centuries of medical practice and scientific discovery. Ancient Indian surgeons, as documented in the *Sushruta Samhita (India)*, 2500 years ago utilized *skin grafting* techniques for wound healing. Over time, critical scientific milestones have reshaped our understanding of the human body and its capacity to heal.

R. D. Arora (✉)
Arora Pain Clinic, Torrance, CA, USA



R. D. Arora (ed.), *Regenerative Medicine in Pain Practice*,
https://doi.org/10.1007/978-3-032-22644-0_1

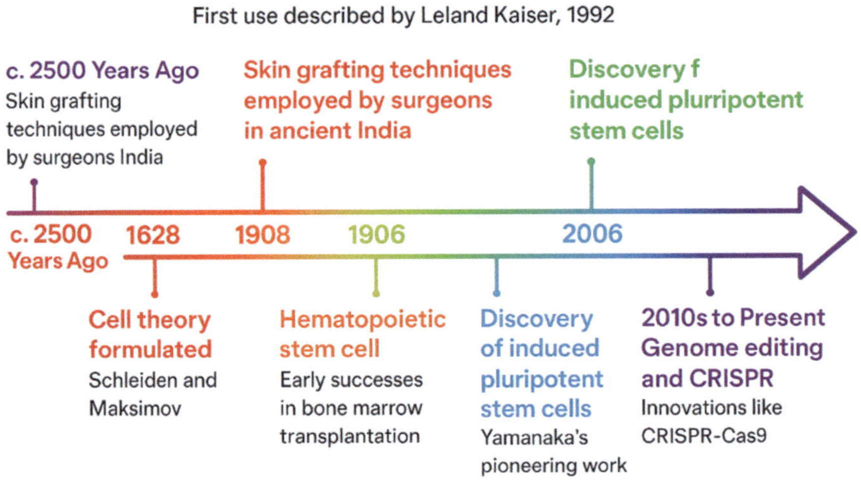


**Fig. 1.1** History of regenerative medicine

**Scientific milestones in progression of regenerative medicine as follows**

- *1628—Discovery of Blood Circulation*
  *William Harvey* described how blood circulates through the body, carrying oxygen, nutrients, and signals. It laid the groundwork for understanding tissue repair.
- *1838—Cell Theory Formulated*
  *Matthias Schleiden and Theodor Schwann* proposed that all living organisms are made of cells, revolutionizing biology and regenerative science.
- *1908—Coining of Term "Stem Cell"*
  *Alexander Maksimov* introduced the concept of "stem cells," recognizing the regenerative potential of undifferentiated cells.

**Modern Regenerative Medicine Milestones**

- *1960s–1980s—Hematopoietic Stem Cell Research*
  Early bone marrow transplantation successes demonstrated the clinical power of stem cells in treating blood disorders.
- *1991—Term "Mesenchymal Stem Cell" (MSC)*
  *Dr. Arnold Caplan* coined this term defining these bone marrow derived cells as having the potential to differentiate into a variety of cell lineages (osteocytes, adipocytes, and chondrocytes). He later advocated for renaming these cells as "Medicinal Signaling Cells" following evidence that showed these cells exert their therapeutic effect by residing in sites of injury and secreting signaling factors with regenerative and immunomodulatory effects.
- *1992—Term "Regenerative Medicine"*
  *Leland Kaiser* formally used the term "regenerative medicine," framing the field as a new branch of medical science.

- *1990s—Human Embryonic Stem Cells*
  *William Haseltine* highlighted embryonic pluripotent cells' ability to differentiate into all cell types.
  *1995–1998*: Human embryonic stem cells and germ cells were first isolated, providing a major leap in regenerative research.
- *1996—Cloning Breakthrough*
  The cloning of *Dolly the sheep* proved that adult cells could be reprogrammed, igniting worldwide interest in cellular plasticity.

**Twenty-First Century Advances**

- *2006—Induced Pluripotent Stem Cells (iPSCs)*
  *Dr. Shinya Yamanaka* developed iPSC technology, reprogramming adult cells into pluripotent ones. This breakthrough earned him the Nobel Prize.
- *2010s–Present—Genome Editing Revolution Occurred*
  CRISPR-Cas9 genome-editing tools allowed precise DNA modifications, opening doors for personalized regenerative medicine.
  - *2020*: *Jennifer Doudna and Emmanuelle Charpentier were* awarded the Nobel Prize for CRISPR-Cas9.
  - *Dec 2023*: FDA approved CRISPR-Cas9 therapy for sickle cell disease, marking the first clinical genome-editing treatment.
  - Ongoing: Research into Down's syndrome genome engineering (reducing trisomy DNA burden).

## 1.3 Evolution

Regenerative medicine has seen remarkable global growth in both scientific research and clinical applications in last decade. This progress reflects a significant shift in healthcare from traditional symptom management toward tissue repair and biologic restoration. As a result, regenerative therapies are becoming increasingly in demand in specialties such as interventional pain management, orthopedics, and sports medicine.

Over the past two decades, research in regenerative medicine and tissue engineering has substantially expanded globally with the United States leading much of the output.

In 2016, there were approximately 30,000 research articles available on this subject (Fig. 1.2). Today, the field is supported by a rapidly growing infrastructure, including hundreds of dedicated journals, conferences, and workshops held annually. Currently, more than 300,000 articles worldwide focus on emerging trends in regenerative medicine. The United States remains a key contributor, alongside other leading countries such as India, Japan, Brazil, and Canada.

*Several factors are responsible for this progress*:

1. Limitations of existing treatments:
   Conventional therapies such as NSAIDs, corticosteroids, opioids, and surgery carry risks ranging from dependency and immunosuppression to tissue

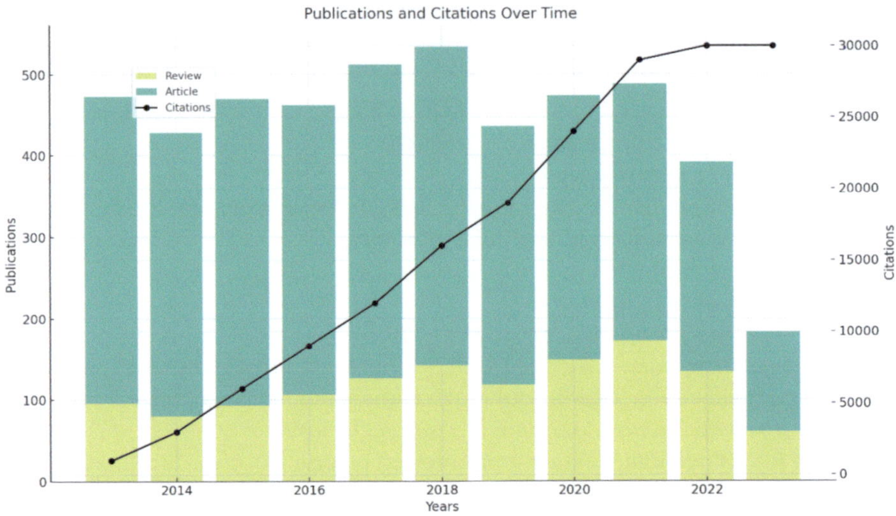


**Fig. 1.2** Progress in research and publications in regenerative medicine and economical trends

degradation and surgical complications. Patients and providers alike are actively seeking alternatives that offer repair, healing, and regeneration rather than just symptom control.

2. Growing clinical data and safety profile:
   PRP and stem cell therapies, initially introduced in sports medicine, have now expanded into mainstream musculoskeletal and spine care, supported by a growing number of randomized controlled trials and systematic reviews.
3. Technological advancements:
   The refinement of biological preparation techniques like improved centrifugation protocols, cellular assays, and exosome isolation has enhanced the efficacy, consistency, and accessibility of regenerative products.
4. Patient demand and awareness:
   Increasingly health-literate patients are asking about biological alternatives. This demand is transforming regenerative medicine from a niche intervention to a sought-after offering in comprehensive clinical pain practices.

This demand is not speculative, it is measurable. Numerous publications and meta-analyses have documented the surge in clinical trials (Fig. 1.3), particularly for applications in osteoarthritis, tendon injuries, rotator cuff tears, meniscal injuries, discogenic back pain, and facet joint arthropathies.

Regenerative medicine is no longer an emerging field; it is a rapidly maturing domain that is redefining standards of care in musculoskeletal and pain medicine. This is an emerging paradigm shift in healthcare. It holds an immense potential to reshape pain medicine by harnessing the body's own healing mechanisms.

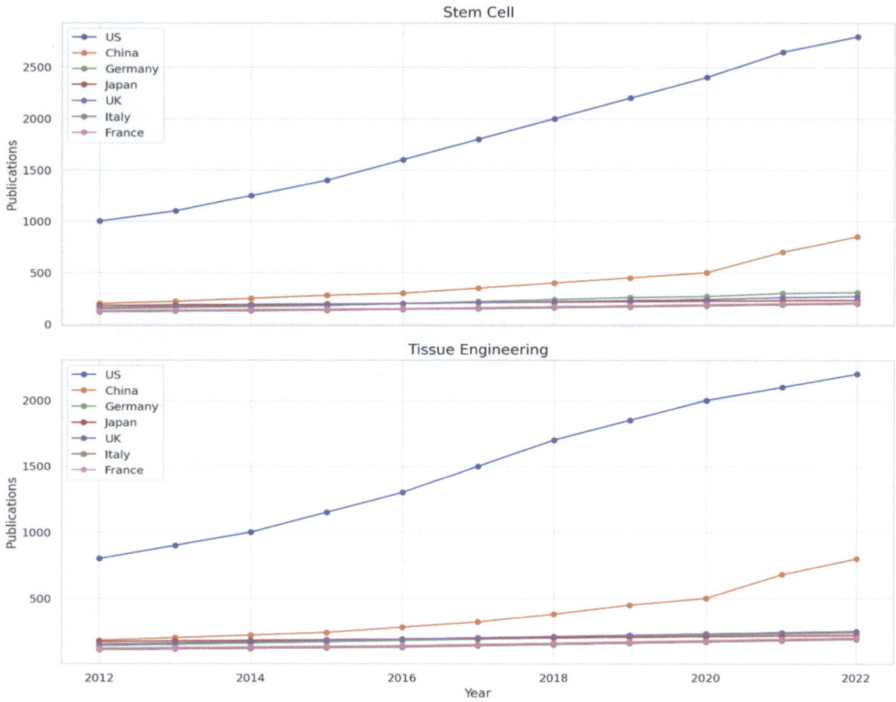


**Fig. 1.3** Progress in research and publications in regenerative medicine and economical trends

## 1.4 Regenerative Medicine Market Growth in the United States

The regenerative medicine market in the United States is experiencing exponential growth, currently valued at approximately $14.5 billion, with projections of $30 billion by 2030, as shown in the graph below (Fig. 1.4).

This upward trend is clearly reflected in leading clinical research centers and biotech companies, where investment in regenerative technologies has accelerated significantly over the past decade. This surge in funding and innovation highlights the growing confidence in regenerative medicine as a transformative force in modern healthcare.

The global regenerative medicine market is expected to grow significantly, fueled by rapid advancements in biotechnology, a rising burden of chronic diseases, and by increased investments in stem cell research and tissue engineering.

Globally, several factors are contributing to this expansion which include strong research capabilities and a well-established healthcare infrastructure, especially in the United States, which takes the lead worldwide. Europe is showing steady growth supported by favorable regulatory frameworks. In the Asia-Pacific

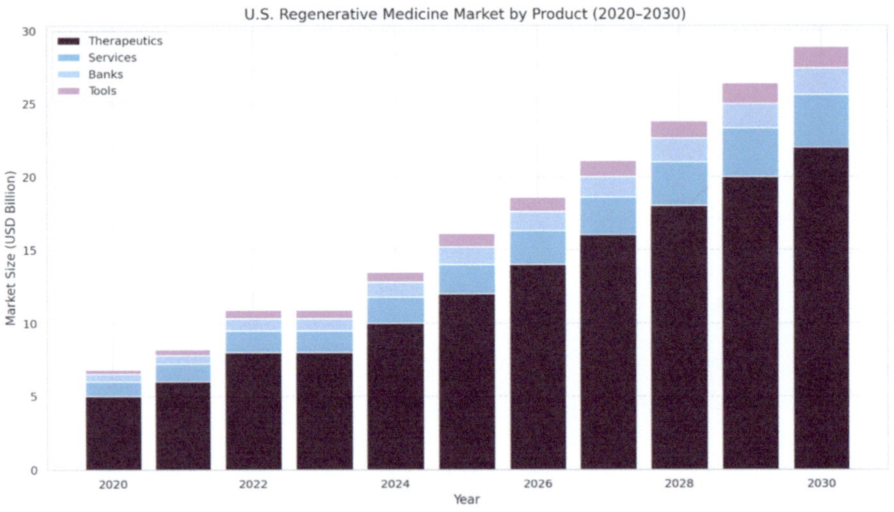


**Fig. 1.4** Progress in research and publications in regenerative medicine and economical trends

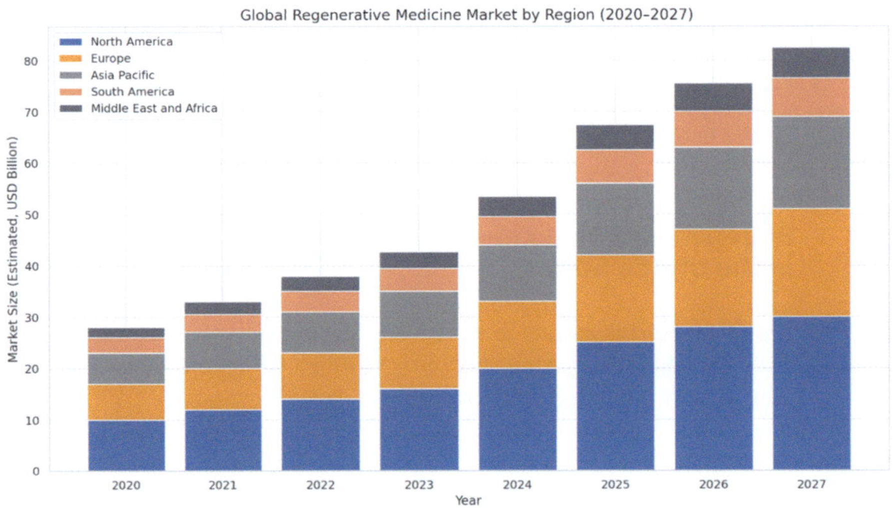


**Fig. 1.5** Progress in research and publications in regenerative medicine and economical trends

region, increasing healthcare spending and innovation are driving progress, and even in South America momentum is gaining through emerging biotech initiatives.

This forecast highlights the global clinical and economic potential of regenerative medicine, with North America and Asia-Pacific anticipated to be the key drivers of growth through 2027 (Fig. 1.5).

# Biology of Tissue Healing and Wound Repair

2

## Hemostasis, Inflammation, Repair, and Regeneration

Ripu D. Arora

Knowledge of the natural pathophysiology of wound healing in the human body and an understanding of the cellular and molecular basis of inflammation and tissue repair is foundational to applying regenerative medicine in a clinical pain practice.

Regeneration is not merely a reversal of damage, it is a well-planned and orchestrated process involving immune modulation, angiogenesis, extracellular matrix remodeling, and cellular differentiation leading to tissue healing.

The physiological response to tissue damage and resultant healing process happens in four phases.

## 2.1 Phases of Normal Tissue Healing

### 2.1.1 Phase of Hemostasis (0–3 h)

The first phase is hemostasis. When there is trauma to the tissues and blood vessels, platelets are released at the site of injury. These platelets contain a special glycoprotein IIb/IIIa called integrin $\alpha_{IIb}\beta_3$ which is responsible for the aggregation of platelets. Once platelets are activated, the discoid cell changes its shape with the formation of pseudopods which help increase the surface area for adhesions by binding fibrinogen and forming bridges between platelets to facilitate aggregation (Fig. 2.1).

During this process vasoconstriction occurs, primarily due to thromboxane and serotonin, which are released by the platelets. Additionally, histamine is released, causing vasodilation around the damaged tissue. This vasodilation leads to the recruitment of hematopoietic cells, various healing substances, and stem cells to the injury site to promote healing.

R. D. Arora (✉)
Arora Pain Clinic, Torrance, CA, USA



R. D. Arora (ed.), *Regenerative Medicine in Pain Practice*,
https://doi.org/10.1007/978-3-032-22644-0_2

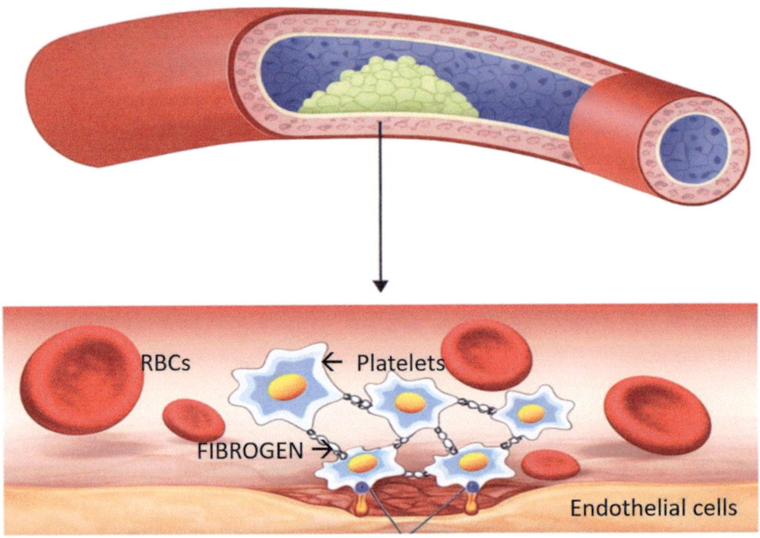


**Fig. 2.1** Discoid platelets with pseudopods undergoing aggregation

*Simultaneously, coagulation factors are released.* Both intrinsic and extrinsic coagulation pathways are activated, leading to the formation of a blood clot.

#### 2.1.1.1 Intrinsic Pathway

This pathway begins when blood contacts negatively charged surfaces like exposed collagen from the damaged endothelium. This triggers a cascade starting with Factor XII, which activates Factor XI, then Factor IX, and in the presence of Factor VIII, leads to the activation of Factor X. This pathway is slower but amplifies the coagulation process and is essential for sustained clot formation.

#### 2.1.1.2 Extrinsic Pathway

This pathway is triggered by external trauma that causes blood to escape the vascular system. It begins with the release of tissue factor (TF), also known as Factor III, from damaged tissues. The tissue factor binds Factor VII, activating it. The TF–VIIa complex then directly activates Factor X. This pathway is rapid and provides the initial "spark" for coagulation.

#### 2.1.1.3 Common Pathway

Once Factor X is activated by either the intrinsic or extrinsic pathway, it combines with Factor V to form the prothrombinase complex. This complex converts prothrombin (Factor II) into thrombin, a key enzyme in clotting. Thrombin then converts fibrinogen (Factor I) into fibrin, which forms a stable meshwork that reinforces the platelet plug. Thrombin also activates Factor XIII, which cross-links fibrin strands, stabilizing the clot and completing the coagulation cascade (Fig. 2.2).

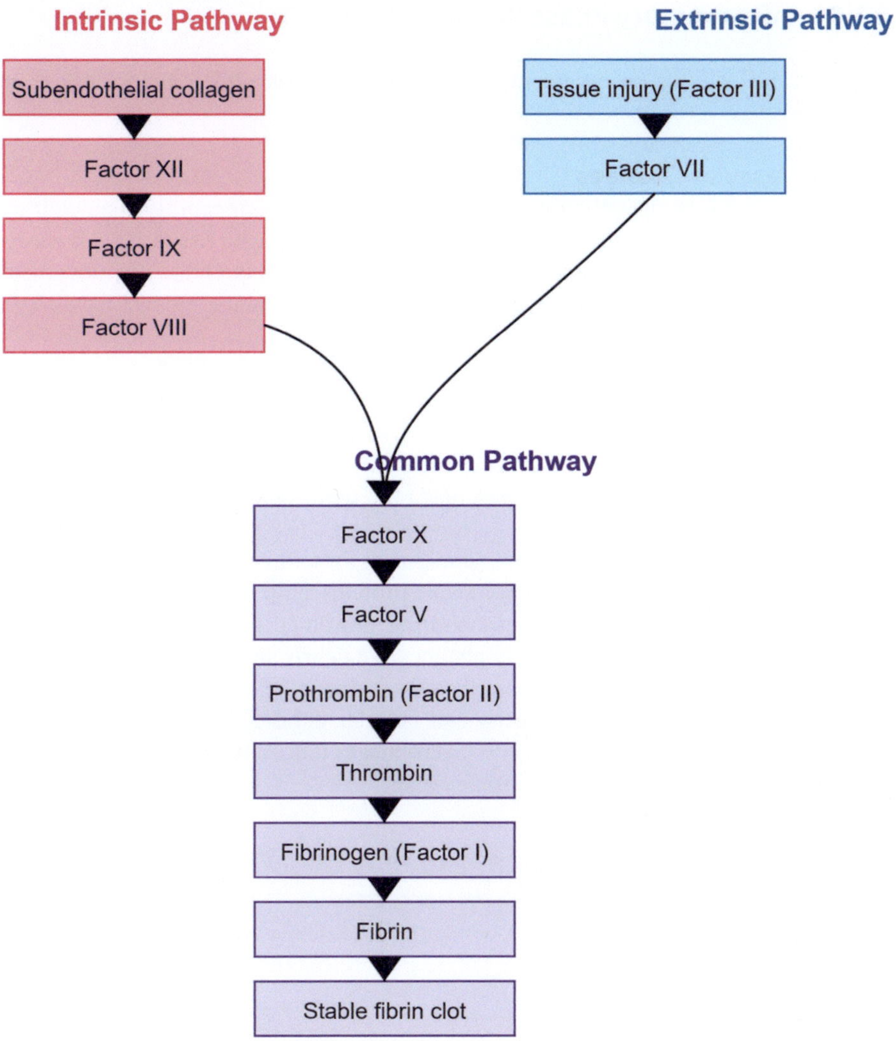


**Fig. 2.2** Clotting cascade

As the fibrin clot forms via the coagulation cascade, the bleeding is effectively stopped.

At the same time, other proteins and chemical signals are also released to support the healing process.

### 2.1.2 Inflammatory Phase (0–7 Days) (Fig. 2.3)

Vascular and cellular events occur simultaneously in the inflammatory phase as follows:

#### 2.1.2.1 Vascular Changes

In response to injury, vasodilation and increased vascular permeability occur, allowing immune cells and plasma proteins to infiltrate the damaged tissue. This is mediated by the release of histamine and prostaglandins, which facilitate the movement of chemical mediators and immune cells into the injured area.

#### 2.1.2.2 Cellular Events

*Arachidonic acid metabolism*: Cell membrane phospholipids are converted into arachidonic acid, which is then acted upon by cyclooxygenase enzymes (COX-1 and COX-2) to form prostaglandin E2 (PGE2), prostacyclin, and thromboxane. These lipid mediators regulate vascular tone, pain, and further recruitment of immune cells.

*Complement system activation*: The complement system is also activated, enhancing the immune response. Complement proteins help form membrane attack complexes to eliminate pathogens and tag unwanted substances for removal. They also stimulate neutrophils to phagocytize debris and pathogens.

*Cellular recruitment*: Neutrophils are the first immune cells to arrive at the injury site, where they engulf pathogens and cellular debris. They are followed by monocytes, which differentiate into macrophages that continue phagocytosis and secrete signaling molecules for tissue repair.

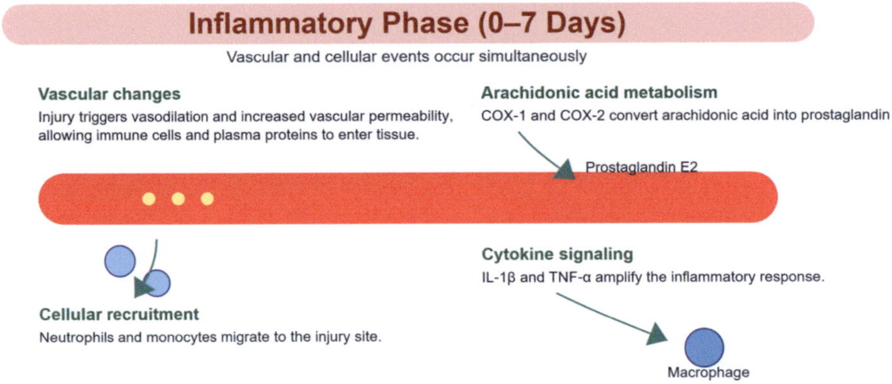


**Fig. 2.3** Illustration of the synchronized vascular and cellular processes that characterize the inflammatory phase of tissue repair. Vasodilation and increased vascular permeability allow plasma proteins and immune cells to infiltrate damaged tissue. Concurrently, arachidonic acid metabolism through COX-1 and COX-2 pathways produces prostaglandins, prostacyclin, and thromboxane, modulating vascular tone and inflammation. Neutrophils and macrophages participate in debris clearance, while cytokines (TNF-α, IL-1β) and complement system activation amplify the immune response and initiate transition to the proliferative phase

*Cytokine signaling*: Interleukin-1β (IL-1β), tumor necrosis factor-alpha (TNF-α), and prostaglandins further shape the local environment by promoting inflammation, recruiting additional immune cells, and initiating the transition to the next phase of healing.

When monocytes leave the bloodstream and enter injured tissue, they differentiate into macrophages. These macrophages can polarize into different functional subtypes, mainly:

**M1 macrophages (classically activated)**
These are pro-inflammatory. They dominate early in the inflammatory phase and are activated by signals such as interferon-gamma (IFN-γ) and lipopolysaccharide (LPS). Their main functions include the following:

- Phagocytosis of pathogens and dead cells
- Production of inflammatory cytokines (e.g., IL-1β, TNF-α, IL-6)
- Recruitment of neutrophils and more immune cells
- Switch from M1 to M2 macrophages

As inflammation begins to resolve, the local environment changes.

Anti-inflammatory signals such as IL-4, IL-10, IL-13, and TGF-β (transforming growth factor) promote the polarization of M1 into M2 macrophages.

**M2 macrophages (alternatively activated)**
These dominate during the proliferative phase and are crucial for tissue repair. Their roles include the following:

- Secretion of anti-inflammatory cytokines (e.g., IL-10, TGF-β)
- Stimulation of angiogenesis via VEGF
- Activation and recruitment of fibroblasts
- Promotion of extracellular matrix (ECM) deposition, especially collagen
- Support for epithelial cell migration and proliferation

The transition is not a binary switch; it is a dynamic spectrum, and the local cytokine milieu and cellular interactions guide this shift.

### 2.1.3 Proliferative Phase (Day 4 to Week 3) (Fig. 2.4)

Once the inflammatory phase subsides, the body shifts to rebuilding tissue.

*Fibroblast activation and collagen synthesis*: Fibroblasts migrate into the wound area and begin producing type III collagen and ECM components to provide a structural framework for new tissue.

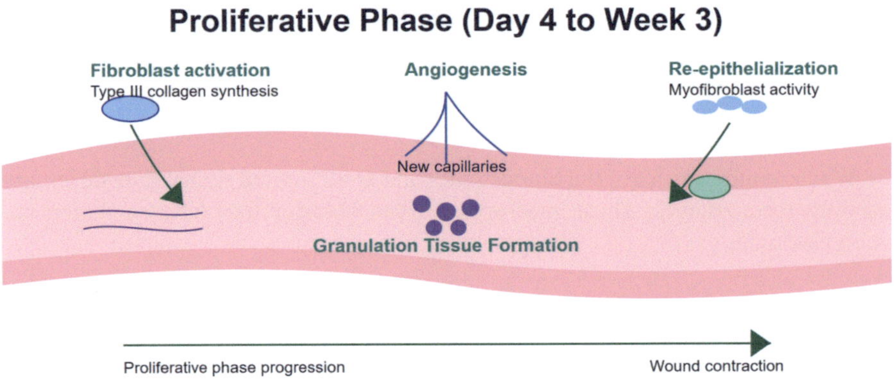


**Fig. 2.4** Proliferative phase

*Angiogenesis*: Stimulated by vascular endothelial growth factor (VEGF) and other signals, new capillaries sprout from existing blood vessels to supply oxygen and nutrients to the healing tissue.

*Granulation tissue formation*: A mix of fibroblasts, new blood vessels, immune cells, and ECM forms granulation tissue, which fills the wound space and supports regeneration.

*Re-epithelialization*: Keratinocytes proliferate and migrate across the wound bed, restoring the epidermal barrier. This is guided by growth factors like epidermal growth factor (EGF) and transforming growth factor-alpha (TGF-α).

*Wound contraction*: Myofibroblasts, modified fibroblasts with contractile ability, pull the edges of the wound together, reducing its size.

#### 2.1.3.1 Role of Fibroblasts in Matrix Formation

Fibroblasts are essential stromal cells activated during the proliferative phase in response to cytokines especially TGF-β and PDGF, chemokines and growth factors released by M2 macrophages, platelets, and damaged cells.

The activated fibroblasts migrate into wounds, proliferate and produce ECM components like type III collagen, fibronectin, hyaluronic acid, and proteoglycans.

Later, fibroblasts help transition the matrix with following events:

- Replace type III collagen with type I collagen, which has greater tensile strength.
- Differentiate into myofibroblasts, contributing to wound contraction through actin-mediated pulling forces.

M2 macrophages and fibroblasts maintain a feedback loop:

- M2 macrophages secrete TGF-β which stimulates fibroblasts.
- Fibroblasts secrete ECM and factors which stabilize tissue and may further suppress inflammation.

### 2.1.4 Remodeling (Maturation) Phase (Fig. 2.5)

This final phase can last for weeks to months, depending on the wound. Events in the final phase are as follows:

*Collagen remodeling*: Type III collagen is gradually replaced by type I collagen, which is stronger and more organized. This improves the tensile strength of the repaired tissue.

*Apoptosis (programmed cell death) of excess cells*: Unneeded fibroblasts, capillaries, and immune cells undergo apoptosis, helping to resolve the hypercellular and hypervascular granulation tissue.

*Scar formation*: A scar forms from dense collagen and ECM, restoring tissue integrity but not necessarily the original function or appearance.

*Vascular regression*: As the metabolic demands of the tissue decrease, many of the new capillaries formed during angiogenesis are resorbed.

### 2.1.5 Summary (Table 2.1) and (Fig. 2.6)

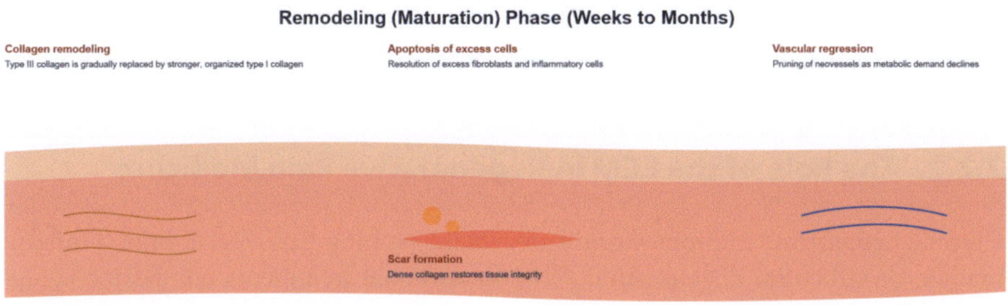


**Fig. 2.5** Remodeling and scar formation

**Table 2.1** Summary

| Phase | Key cell types | Functions |
|---|---|---|
| Early inflammation | M1 macrophages | Clear pathogens and debris, secrete pro-inflammatory cytokines |
| Proliferation | M2 macrophages | Anti-inflammatory, promote fibroblast activity and ECM formation |
| Matrix formation | Fibroblasts and myofibroblasts | Produce ECM (collagen, fibronectin), remodel tissue, contract wound |

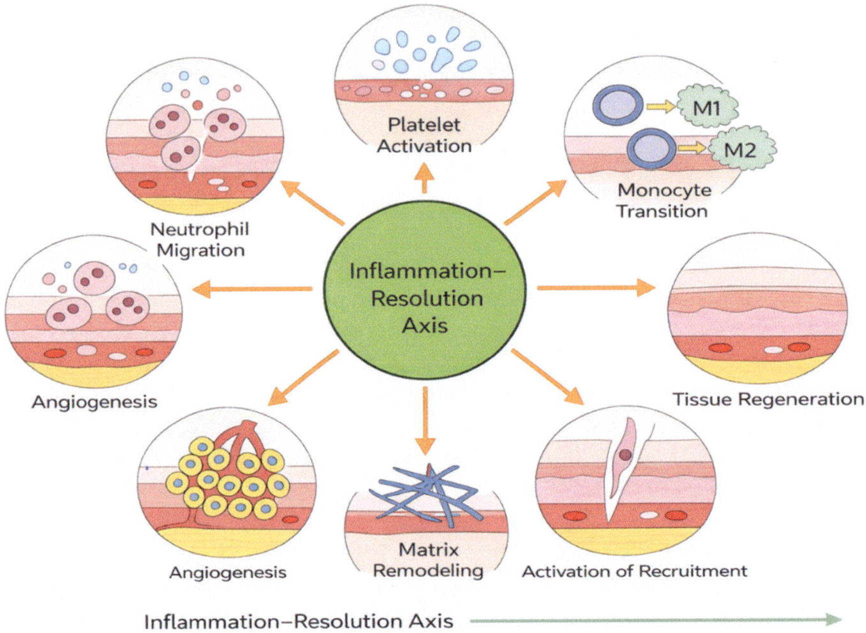


**Fig. 2.6** Summary of regenerative process

## 2.2 The Role of the ECM in Regenerative Pain Medicine

Chronic pain affects millions worldwide, often resulting from tissue injury, inflammation, or structural degeneration. While traditional treatments emphasize symptom control through pharmacologic or interventional methods, regenerative medicine targets the root cause of pain by promoting tissue repair and functional restoration. Central to this regenerative approach is the ECM, a dynamic and biologically active scaffold that influences nearly every aspect of tissue development, maintenance, and healing.

The ECM is a complex, three-dimensional network composed of proteins and carbohydrates, including collagens, elastin, proteoglycans, glycoproteins, and growth factors.

Far beyond a passive scaffold, the ECM is an active participant in regulating cell behavior, such as cell adhesion, proliferation, differentiation, migration, and apoptosis (Fig. 2.7).

These processes are essential for tissue integrity, injury response, and regeneration, making the ECM a critical focus in regenerative pain therapy.

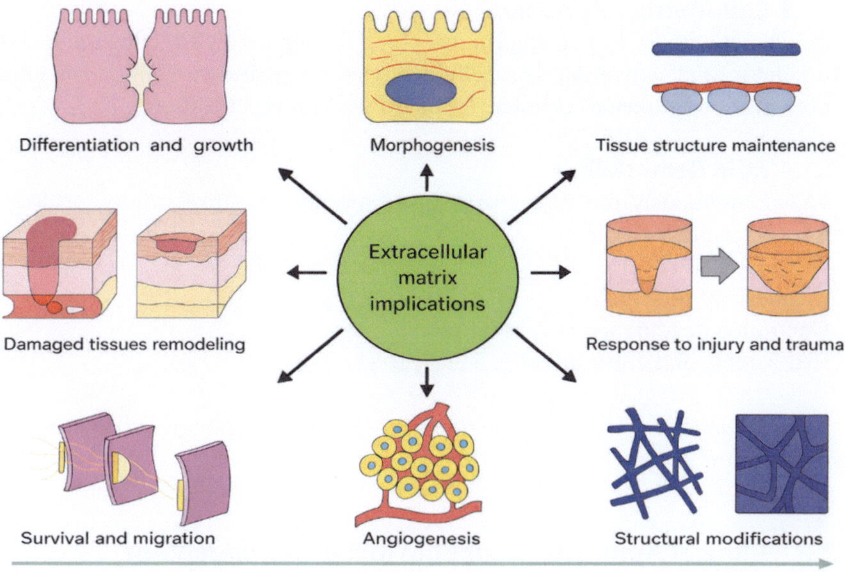


**Fig. 2.7** Role of ECM

## 2.2.1 How ECM Is Formed

### 2.2.1.1 Cellular Synthesis of ECM Components

ECM is synthesized primarily by resident cells within each tissue type, for example:

Fibroblasts in connective tissues
Chondrocytes in cartilage
Osteoblasts in bone
Smooth muscle and endothelial cells in blood vessels
Epithelial cells in skin

*The synthesized components include the following*:

Structural Proteins: Collagen (strength), elastin (elasticity)
Adhesive Glycoproteins: Fibronectin, laminin
Proteoglycans: Hyaluronic acid, chondroitin sulfate

### 2.2.1.2 Secretion and Extracellular Assembly

Components are secreted via exocytosis and assemble into structured networks in the extracellular space. Enzymes such as lysyl oxidase facilitate cross-linking, while matrix metalloproteinases (MMPs) remodel the matrix during growth or repair.

#### 2.2.1.3 Cell-Matrix Interaction

Cells interact with ECM via integrin receptors, linking the ECM to the intracellular cytoskeleton and activating intracellular signaling pathways. This bidirectional communication influences cellular responses vital for regeneration.

#### 2.2.1.4 ECM Remodeling

ECM is continuously remodeled to adapt to mechanical stress, injury, or disease. This involves the following:

- Synthesis of new ECM
- Controlled degradation (via MMPs)
- Reassembly and cross-linking

*An imbalance in this remodeling process contributes to pathological pain states, such as fibrosis or degeneration.*

### 2.2.2 Clinical Applications of ECM in Pain Management

The principles of ECM biology are now applied in several regenerative pain therapies:

### 2.2.3 Summary (Table 2.2)

The ECM is the master regulator of tissue regeneration. It orchestrates cell behavior, supports structural integrity, and initiates repair mechanisms crucial for resolving pain at its source. In regenerative medicine, ECM-based strategies enable tissue-specific healing that goes beyond symptomatic relief to achieve functional restoration and long-term pain resolution (Table 2.2).

As clinical science continues to uncover the full potential of ECM, its integration into pain management represents a powerful evolution in personalized, biologically grounded care.

**Table 2.2** Applications of ECM

| Application area | ECM-based approach |
|---|---|
| Osteoarthritis | ECM-rich hydrogels, stem cells on ECM scaffolds |
| Tendinopathies | ECM patches, PRP with ECM-derived cytokines |
| Degenerative disc disease | ECM-injected biomaterials, peptide-based matrix enhancers |
| Peripheral neuropathy | ECM conduits, nerve wrap products |
| Post-surgical pain | ECM implants to reduce fibrosis and adhesions |

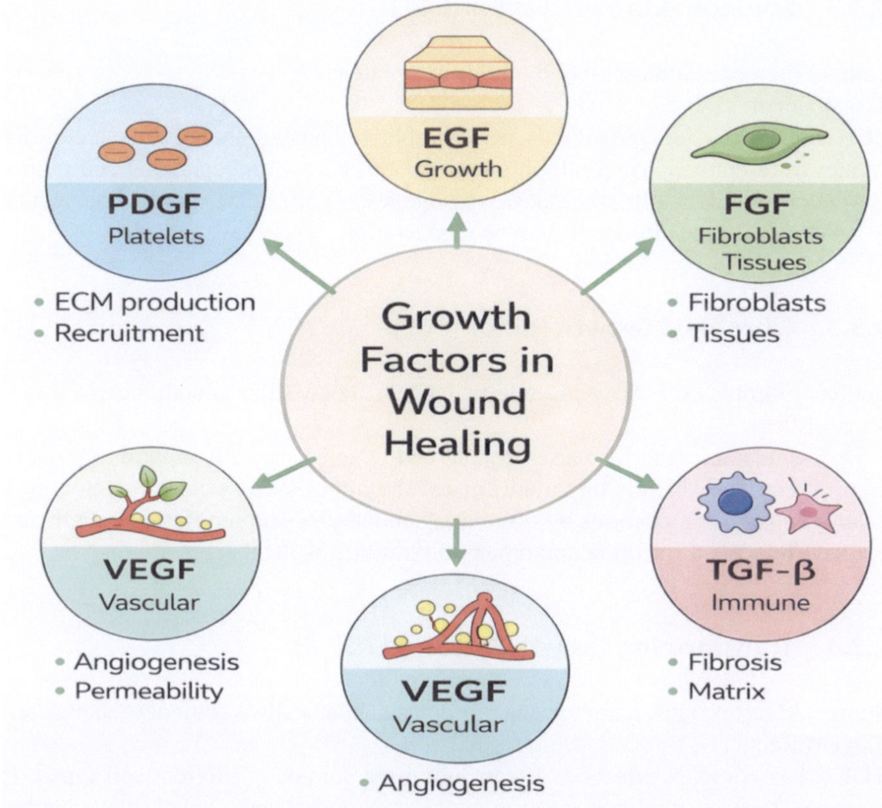


**Fig. 2.8** Growth factors involved in tissue regeneration

## 2.3 Growth Factors in Tissue Repair and Regeneration

*The growth factors involved in repair of tissues released from platelets and other cells are listed below* (Fig. 2.8):

### 2.3.1 Platelet-Derived Growth Factor (PDGF)

Source: Endothelial cells, platelets, macrophages, fibroblasts
Target/Effect:
PDGF is mitogenic (stimulates cell division) for vascular smooth muscle cells and fibroblasts. It plays a critical role in the early stages of wound healing by recruiting neutrophils, macrophages, and fibroblasts to the injury site and by stimulating fibroblast proliferation and migration. It also enhances collagen production and matrix formation.

### 2.3.2 Epidermal Growth Factor (EGF)

Source: Present in almost all body fluids and platelets
Target/Effect:
EGF is mitogenic for epithelial tissues, fibroblasts, and endothelial cells. It contributes to re-epithelialization by promoting keratinocyte and epithelial cell migration/proliferation. It stimulates angiogenesis and ECM production which enhances wound closure and tissue regeneration.

### 2.3.3 Fibroblast Growth Factor (FGF)

Source: Fibroblasts, astrocytes, endothelial cells, bone cells, smooth muscle
Target/Effect:
FGF acts as a mitogen for mesenchymal and neural tissues. It supports fibroblast proliferation, which is important for ECM synthesis and wound contraction. It also helps in angiogenesis by stimulating endothelial cell proliferation. FGF also plays important role in neural repair and musculoskeletal regeneration.

### 2.3.4 Transforming Growth Factor-β (TGF-β)

Source: Macrophages, lymphocytes, fibroblasts, bone cells, keratinocytes, platelets
Target/Effect:
TGF-β has complex effects as it can inhibit or stimulate different cell types. In wound healing, it inhibits replication of keratinocytes, endothelial cells, lymphocytes, and macrophages in vitro. It regulates fibroblast activity, stimulating collagen synthesis and matrix deposition, which plays a key role in scar formation and immune modulation. It is also critical for M2 macrophage polarization and transition from inflammation to repair.

### 2.3.5 Vascular Endothelial Growth Factor (VEGF)

Source: Pituitary cells (though also widely expressed in other tissues during wound healing)
Target/Effect:
VEGF is specifically mitogenic for endothelial cells, but not for keratinocytes, smooth muscle, or fibroblasts. It is crucial for angiogenesis by promoting the growth of new blood vessels into the healing tissue. This improves oxygen and nutrient delivery to the regenerating area. It supports survival and function of newly formed capillaries.

# Regenerative Therapies for Pain Practice 3

Ripu D. Arora

Regenerative therapies (e.g., platelet-rich plasma, stem cell-based treatments, growth factors, exosome and other biologics) aim to reprogram the inflammatory environment from a chronic, destructive, degenerative state to a pro-resolution, repair, and pro-regenerative state.

## 3.1 Acute Inflammation to Chronic Dysfunction Process

Acute inflammation serves as a critical trigger for tissue repair, mobilizing immune cells, clearing debris, and initiating regeneration. This tightly regulated response is essential for normal wound healing.

However, in chronic pain syndromes such as osteoarthritis, chronic tendinopathy, and discogenic back pain the inflammatory process becomes low-grade, persistent, and maladaptive. Instead of resolving, inflammation remains smoldering and causes continued tissue degradation, impaired healing, and sensitization of nociceptive pathways, contributing to chronic pain.

## 3.2 Factors Responsible for Degeneration

*The factors responsible for degeneration include the following*:

Persistent activation of macrophages (often M1-dominant)
Ongoing release of pro-inflammatory cytokines (e.g., IL-6, TNF-α)
Matrix breakdown and fibrosis, dysregulation of remodeling (MMPs)

R. D. Arora (✉)
Arora Pain Clinic, Torrance, CA, USA



R. D. Arora (ed.), *Regenerative Medicine in Pain Practice*,
https://doi.org/10.1007/978-3-032-22644-0_3

## 3.3 Goals of Regenerative Therapies

*The goals of regenerative therapies include the following*:

1. Restore tissue homeostasis and function
2. Promote a shift from M1 to M2 macrophage phenotypes
3. Stimulate angiogenesis and matrix synthesis
4. Downregulate pro-inflammatory cytokines
5. Encourage the recruitment of endogenous stem cells
6. Correct the immune imbalance: immunomodulation

Regenerative therapies offer not just symptom relief, but also the potential for true tissue regeneration, especially in conditions where healing has failed due to ongoing inflammation.

## 3.4 Orthobiologics

*Available orthobiologics are as follows*:

*Autograft*:
  Bone marrow adult stem cells
  Adipose (fat) tissue adult mesenchymal stem cells
  Platelet-rich plasma
*Allograft*:
  Umbilical cord tissue and blood
  Amniotic tissue and fluids
*Xenograft*:
  From different species (not used in humans)

## 3.5 Different Cell Products (Fig. 3.1)

### 3.5.1 Adult Stem Cells

*Mesenchymal Stem Cells (MSCs)*: Found in bone marrow, adipose tissue, and other sites. Known for their potential to differentiate into bones, cartilage, and fat cells.

*Hematopoietic Stem Cells (HSCs)*: Adult hematopoiesis occurs in red bone marrow. HSCs are primarily responsible for generating blood cell lineages.

*Neonatal-Derived Stem Cells*: Harvested from umbilical cord blood or tissue.

These cells are used in other regenerative therapies (e.g., bone marrow aspirate concentrate, stem cell injections), but they are not present in PRP, which is derived purely from peripheral blood.

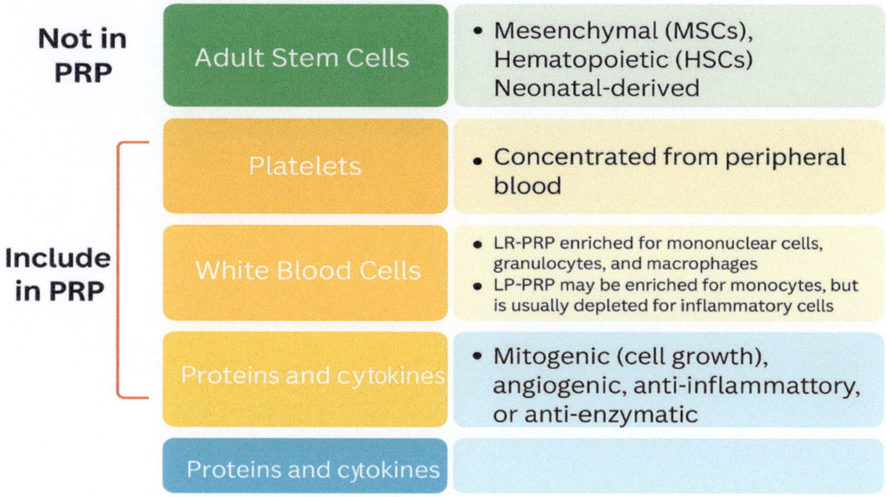


**Fig. 3.1** Different cell products in PRP and BMA

### 3.5.2 Platelet-Rich Plasma (PRP)

*Source*: Concentrated from peripheral blood using centrifugation.

*Function*: Release growth factors and cytokines that help in healing, tissue regeneration, and reducing inflammation. The cytokines and proteins, biomolecules which are bioactive compounds in PRP, are responsible for its healing properties such as:

- *Mitogenic*: Promote cell proliferation and repair.
- *Angiogenic*: Stimulate blood vessel formation, essential for oxygen/nutrient delivery.
- *Anti-inflammatory*: Modulate immune response to minimize pain and swelling.
- *Anti-enzymatic*: Protect tissues by inhibiting enzymes that degrade extracellular matrix (like MMPs in joints).

PRP can be prepared with or without white blood cells producing two subtypes

*LR-PRP (Leukocyte-Rich PRP)*: Contains mononuclear cells, granulocytes, and macrophages. It may induce a stronger inflammatory response and is used where immune activity is beneficial (e.g., infections or tough-to-heal tissues).

*LP-PRP (Leukocyte-Poor PRP)*: May still have monocytes, but it is generally depleted of inflammatory multinucleated cells, making it better for joints or areas where inflammation is undesirable.

Regenerative medicine provides tailored, tissue-specific treatments that bridge the gap between conservative care and surgery. With the use of autologous biologics, many patients can experience pain relief, functional recovery, and delay or avoid invasive interventions.

# 4 Platelet-Rich Plasma (PRP) in Musculoskeletal Conditions

Ripu D. Arora

Platelet-rich plasma (PRP) is an autologous blood product enriched with concentrated platelets, associated cytokines, and growth factors, proposed to promote tissue healing and modulate inflammation.

It has been increasingly utilized in the past two decades as a biologic therapy in various musculoskeletal disorders, particularly for osteoarthritis and tendinopathies.

Platelets are formed from megakaryocytes derived from bone marrow. Each megakaryocyte produces 1000 platelets. Platelets have a life span of 7–10 days.

Activated platelets release platelet growth factors and adhesion molecules that mediate a variety of cellular interactions including chemotaxis, cell adhesion, cell differentiation, and immunomodulatory activities. Activated platelet cell-cell interactions contribute to angiogenesis and inflammatory activities, ultimately stimulating tissue repair processes.

## 4.1 Types of Platelet Granules and Their Functional Roles (Fig. 4.1)

Platelets are small, anucleate cell fragments that play a central role not only in hemostasis but also in tissue regeneration and repair. Their ability to store and release bioactive molecules is made possible by the presence of specialized storage organelles known as granules. These are broadly classified into three types: alpha granules, delta (dense) granules, and lambda granules. Each granule type has a distinct molecular composition and function, contributing to hemostatic, angiogenic, and immunomodulatory processes.

R. D. Arora (✉)
Arora Pain Clinic, Torrance, CA, USA



R. D. Arora (ed.), *Regenerative Medicine in Pain Practice*,
https://doi.org/10.1007/978-3-032-22644-0_4

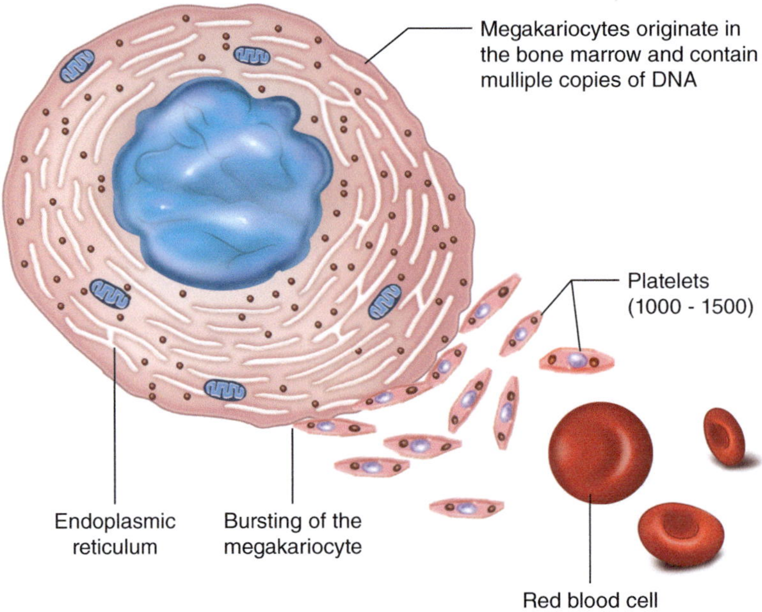


**Fig. 4.1** Platelet-driven cellular signaling and chemokine driven immune cell recruitment for tissue repair

### 4.1.1 Alpha Granules: Reservoir of Growth Factors

- *Composition*: Alpha granules are the most abundant platelet granules, containing over 300 different proteins. These include growth factors, adhesion molecules, cytokines, and chemokines.
- *Key Molecules*: Platelet-derived growth factor (PDGF), vascular endothelial growth factor (VEGF), transforming growth factor-β (TGF-β), insulin-like growth factor (IGF-1), epidermal growth factor (EGF), platelet factor 4 (PF4), fibrinogen, von Willebrand factor, and fibronectin.
- *Functions*:
  - *Wound Healing and Regeneration*: Release of PDGF, VEGF, and TGF-β stimulates angiogenesis, fibroblast proliferation, and extracellular matrix synthesis.
  - *Cell Recruitment*: Chemokines such as PF4 affect stem cells and RANTES attracts stem cells, immune cells, and endothelial progenitor cells to the site of injury.
  - *Tissue Repair*: Growth factors are released to support cell proliferation, differentiation, and remodeling of damaged tissue.

### 4.1.2 Delta (Dense) Granules: Initiators of the Clotting Cascade

- *Composition*: Delta granules contain small, non-protein molecules critical for hemostasis and platelet activation.
- *Key Molecules*: Adenosine diphosphate (ADP), adenosine triphosphate (ATP), calcium ions, serotonin (5-HT), and polyphosphates.
- *Functions*:
  - *Platelet Aggregation*: ADP and ATP act as potent agonists that activate surrounding platelets, amplifying clot formation.
  - *Hemostatic Plug Formation*: Calcium ions are essential cofactors in the coagulation cascade, promoting fibrin formation and stabilization of the platelet plug.
  - *Vascular Constriction*: Serotonin (5-HT) induces vasoconstriction, limiting blood loss at the injury site.
  - *Clot Stabilization*: Polyphosphates enhance thrombin generation and fibrin cross-linking, strengthening the clot.

### 4.1.3 Lambda Granules: Lysosomal Organelles

- *Composition*: Lambda granules, also known as lysosomes, contain hydrolytic enzymes that aid in the breakdown of biomolecules and in the clearance of debris.
- *Key Molecules*: Acid hydrolases, cathepsins, glycosidases, and other degradative enzymes.
- *Functions*:
  - *Clot Remodeling*: Enzymes degrade extracellular matrix components contributing to clot resolution and wound remodeling.
  - *Debris Clearance*: Facilitate the breakdown of cellular fragments and necrotic material at the injury site.
  - *Immunomodulation*: Release of enzymes influences inflammatory pathways, balancing tissue repair and immune response (Fig. 4.2).

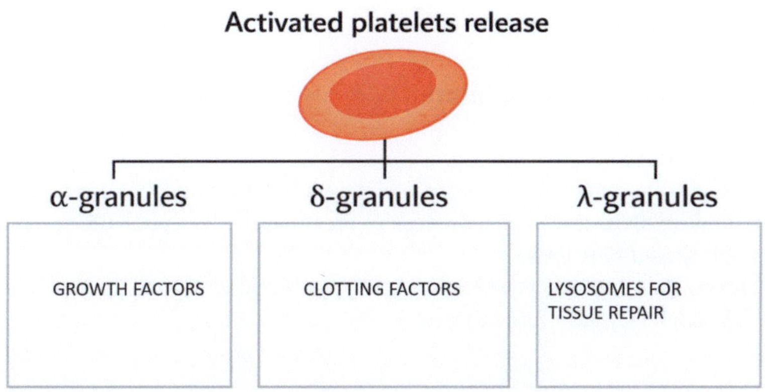


**Fig. 4.2** Granules in activated platelets that release growth factors and cytokines

## 4.2 Preparation of PRP

PRP is prepared through a process of centrifugation, which separates whole blood into its constituent components based on density:

### 4.2.1 Step 1: Blood Collection

The procedure is initiated with the collection of either whole blood or bone marrow aspirate (BMA). This biological sample contains a complex mixture of:

Red blood cells (RBCs), white blood cells (WBCs), platelets and plasma (rich in proteins)
The whole blood is drawn into anticoagulant-treated tubes to prevent clotting.

### 4.2.2 Step 2: Centrifugation

There are two main approaches to centrifugation:

#### 4.2.2.1 Traditional (Hard Spin) Centrifugation

Speed: Greater than 1500× *g*
Time: More than 10 min
Purpose: Maximizes separation of cellular components
This method results in the formation of distinct layers:

- Platelet-Poor Plasma (top layer): Contains plasma proteins but no cells
- Leukocyte-Rich PRP Buffy Coat (middle layer): Rich in platelets and white blood cells (WBCs)
  - When derived from BMA, this layer also contains stem cells, making it a potential source for regenerative applications
- Red Blood Cell Layer (bottom layer): Densest component, not typically used in PRP preparations

This approach produces leukocyte-rich PRP (LR-PRP) or bone marrow concentrate (BMC) with stem cells.

#### 4.2.2.2 Soft Spin Centrifugation

Speed: Lower G-force
Time: Shorter duration
Purpose: Gentle separation to retain platelets while reducing WBC content
This method involves a two-step process to create leukocyte-poor PRP (LP-PRP):

- *Step (a): Initial Soft Spin*
  - The goal of this step is to begin stratifying blood components gently:
    - Plasma "Cloud" (upper layer):

Contains most of the platelets, essential plasma proteins
No WBCs—they remain in the lower layer
LP-PRP Buffy Coat (middle layer):
Reduced in WBCs with some residual platelets

At this point, the platelet-poor plasma can be extracted from the plasma "cloud" to proceed to the next step.

*Step (b): Secondary Centrifugation*

A second round of centrifugation further refines the LP-PRP:
Platelet-Poor Plasma (top layer):
Contains proteins, but no cells
LP-PRP Concentrate (lower layer):
Contains platelets and a few WBCs

The final product is a leukocyte-poor PRP with a high platelet concentration and minimal inflammatory cells (WBCs), ideal for sensitive tissue injections like tendons or joints.

*The blood is spun to yield three distinct layers* (Fig. 4.3a):

Plasma (Top Layer)—~54% of the total volume
It contains water, nutrients, proteins, electrolytes, and metabolic waste.
Buffy Coat (Middle Layer)—~1% of the volume
Rich in white blood cells (neutrophils, monocytes, lymphocytes, etc.) and platelets.
Red Blood Cells (Bottom Layer)—~45% of the volume
Composed of erythrocytes, usually discarded during PRP preparation.

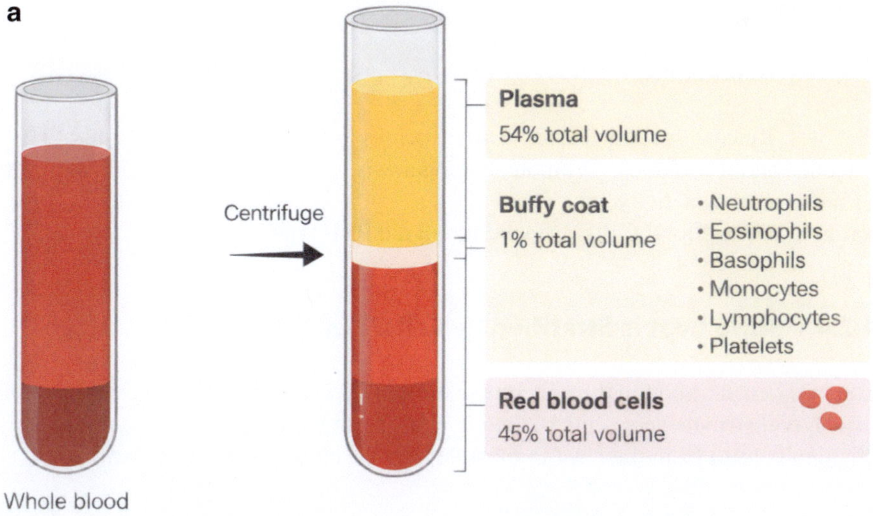


**Fig. 4.3** (**a**) Layers of centrifuged blood . (**b**) Centrifuge second spin for LP-PRP

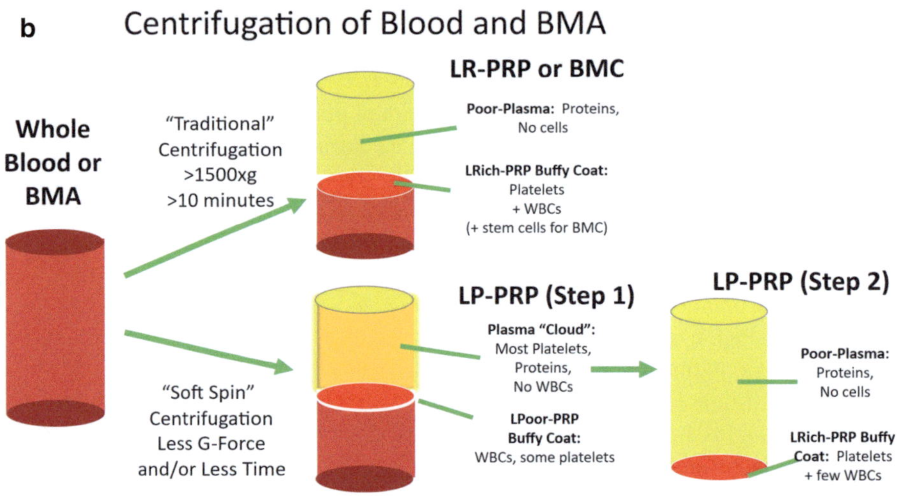


**Fig. 4.3** (continued)

### 4.2.3 Step 3: PRP Collection

PRP can be prepared as in Fig. 4.3b

Leukocyte-Rich PRP (LR-PRP)—includes buffy coat for enhanced immunologic activity.
Leukocyte-Poor PRP (LP-PRP)—avoids buffy coat to reduce pro-inflammatory cell content.

Components of PRP:

Platelets: Release several growth factors such as PDGF, TGF-β, VEGF, and EGF.
Proteins and Cytokines: Promote angiogenesis, cellular proliferation, and anti-inflammatory activity.
Variable White Blood Cells: Depending on the PRP type.

### 4.2.4 Buffy Coat Is Stratified by Cell Density (Fig. 4.4)

The buffy coat, although thin, is compositionally complex. Cellular elements within this layer distribute according to their density, forming a vertical gradient (shown in diagram below) from the least to most dense. The cells are arranged as follows:

Platelets (~1.04–1.06 g/mL): Small, anucleate cell fragments essential for clotting and tissue regeneration. Being least dense, platelets form the top of the buffy coat gradient.

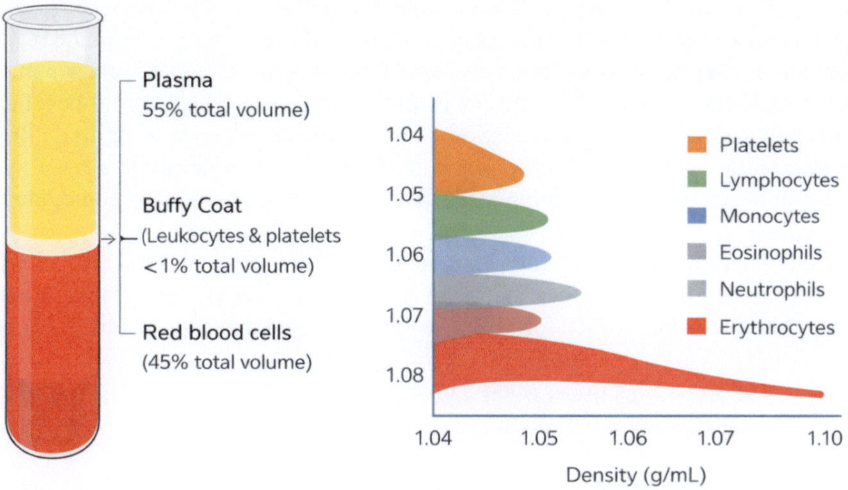


**Fig. 4.4** Layers of cells as per density

Monocytes and Lymphocytes (~1.06–1.08 g/mL): Mononuclear cells with significant roles in immune modulation and tissue healing.

Basophils, Neutrophils, Eosinophils (~1.08–1.09+ g/mL): Multi-nucleated, granulocytic cells often associated with inflammation.

Erythrocytes (~1.10 g/mL): The heaviest component, rich in hemoglobin, forming the base layer.

#### 4.2.4.1 Clinical Considerations in Buffy Coat Harvesting

Two strategic approaches are commonly considered during the harvesting process of the buffy coat, each with distinct clinical implications:

Capturing the *entire buffy coat* maximizes platelet yield. However, it also includes denser, multi-nucleated white blood cells (e.g., neutrophils), which can drive pro-inflammatory responses, and small amounts of RBCs due to their proximity.

This may be more suitable for conditions requiring a more robust inflammatory stimulus (e.g., tendon injuries in early healing stages).

Harvesting only the *upper half of the buffy coat* yields a high concentration of platelets and mononuclear cells (monocytes, lymphocytes), while minimizing inclusion of inflammatory granulocytes, although it has slightly reduced total platelet count. This approach is preferred for chronic pain syndromes or inflammatory conditions (e.g., osteoarthritis) where minimizing inflammation is key.

Depending on the specific goals of the treatment, either leukocyte-rich (LR) or leukocyte-poor (LP) PRP can be prepared through variations in centrifugation speed and time.

For leukocyte-poor PRP, with low numbers of inflammatory WBCs, the primary cells included are T cells and monocytes. These cells contribute to immune regulation and healing through the release of anti-inflammatory cytokines and support of tissue remodeling. While not always essential, their presence is often beneficial, especially in cases where modulation of the immune response is desired. Target concentration is typically less than 5× the baseline. Maintaining this level helps avoid unnecessary inflammation while still leveraging their immunomodulatory properties.

Leukocyte-rich PRP, has high numbers of inflammatory WBCs. Included are neutrophils and macrophages, which are typically associated with acute inflammation. Their inclusion in PRP formulations is conditional and site specific:

For joint or spine injections, a low concentration (0–1X baseline) is preferred to avoid exacerbating inflammation.

For tendon or muscle injuries, a moderate elevation (3–5X baseline) may be beneficial, as these cells can enhance the early inflammatory phase of healing within these tissues. The cellular and molecular composition of whole blood/BMA with their concentrated counterparts, platelet-rich plasma (PRP) and bone marrow concentrate (BMC) differ and each has its own clinical relevance (Fig. 4.5).

### 4.2.5 Red Blood Cells (RBCs) in PRP

Red blood cells (RBCs), or erythrocytes, are anucleate cells primarily responsible for oxygen transport due to their hemoglobin (Hb) content, which forms an iron-containing protein complex. With a lifespan of approximately 120 days, RBCs circulate throughout the body, delivering oxygen to tissues and removing carbon dioxide.

RBCs are cleared by macrophages in the liver and spleen. The hemoglobin break down products of Hemin, free iron, and plasma-free hemoglobin causes cytotoxicity, depletes nitric oxide, and causes eryptosis (inflammatory signaling). The

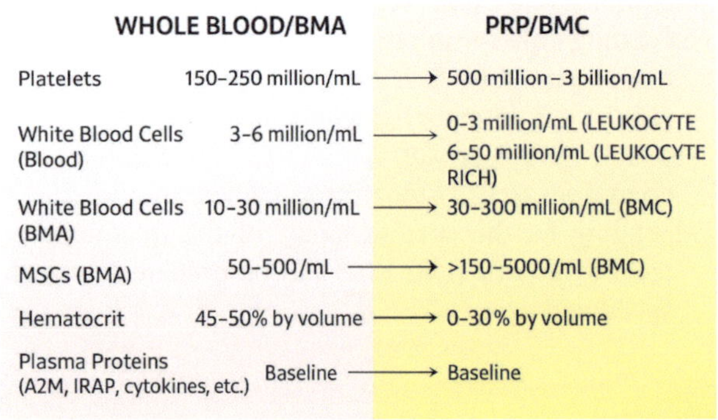


**Fig. 4.5** Comparative cell concentrations in blood-derived biologic therapies

consequences of eryptosis include pro-inflammatory signaling, endothelial damage, loss of vasodilatory nitric oxide, and tissue injury, each of which inhibit stem cell proliferation and fibroblast activity.

In conclusion, RBCs have no known regenerative role in PRP therapy and are generally regarded as undesirable contaminants. Their presence can lead to increased local tissue irritation or toxicity. Therefore, the target concentration for RBCs is 0–1X baseline. Most modern PRP preparation techniques strive to eliminate them completely from the final injectable product.

## 4.3 PRP Types by Volumes and Concentrate

Clinically, we aim for platelets concentration of 1–1.5 billion platelets per milliliter, which represents a 4–8X increase over baseline blood levels. Concentrations above 3 billion/mL may be counterproductive, as some in vitro studies suggest excessively high platelet counts can impair healing, possibly due to overactivation or excessive cytokine release (Table 4.1).

Plasma-soluble factors are important bioactive proteins and anti-inflammatory mediators such as alpha-2-macroglobulin (A2M) and interleukin-1 receptor antagonist protein (IRAP). These components are valuable across various PRP applications for their roles in reducing inflammation and supporting tissue repair. Our goal is for a 5–10X increase in concentration of these soluble factors to maximize their therapeutic benefit in regenerative treatments.

Total platelet count and concentration are important differing therapeutic concepts. High concentration (Super Concentrate) means more platelets per mL, but the total dose (absolute platelet number) can still be matched or exceeded by using a large volume PRP technique.

Large volume PRP has lower concentration of platelets per mL compared to using a Super Concentrate, but it still maintains a high total platelet number because of the larger volume used.

Injections into small anatomical spaces (e.g., wrist joint, TMJ, or the plantar fascia) benefit from using a Super Concentrate PRP, which delivers a potent dose in a small fluid volume.

Super Concentrate PRP contains a higher concentration of plasma-derived bioactive proteins, such as A2M, IRAP (Interleukin-1 Receptor Antagonist Protein),

**Table 4.1** Different PRP types by volume, concentration, as well as composition available for joint use depending on the pathology being treated

| PRP type | Volume (mL) | Platelet/mL (enrichment factor) | Total platelets | Plasma proteins (volume) |
|---|---|---|---|---|
| Super Concentrate | 1 | 4 billion/mL (**20×**) | 4 billion | <1 mL |
| Low volume | 3 | 1.5 billion/mL (**7.5×**) | 4.5 billion | 2–3 mL |
| Typical PRP | 6 | 1 billion/mL (**5×**) | 6 billion | 5 mL |
| Large volume | 10 | 750 million/mL (**3.5×**) | 7.5 billion | 7–8 mL |

**Table 4.2** Matching PRP biologic targets to clinical use

| Biologic factor | Do we want it? | Target concentration | Comments |
|---|---|---|---|
| Platelets | Yes | 1–1.5 billion/mL (4–8x) | >3 billion/mL may be detrimental (in vitro data) |
| Low-inflammatory WBCs | Usually, | <5x | T cells and monocytes support immunomodulation |
| High-inflammatory WBCs | Sometimes | Joints/Spine: 0–1x Tendon/Muscle: 3–5x | Neutrophils/macrophages may increase inflammation |
| Plasma-soluble factors | Yes | 5–10x | Source of A2M, IRAP, and anti-inflammatory cytokines |
| Red blood cells | No | 0–1x | No known regenerative benefit; possible toxicity |

and other anti-inflammatory cytokines per mL than large volume PRP. Generally, a higher concentration means more proteins per volume.

Conclusion: Understanding and selecting the appropriate centrifugation technique is essential for tailoring PRP or BMC to the specific clinical need. While LR-PRP or BMC is ideal for promoting cell regeneration and immune responses, LP-PRP offers a cleaner product suited for reducing inflammation and pain with minimal immune stimulation.

## 4.4 Platelet Poor Plasma

Adding platelet-poor plasma (PPP) can be viewed not just as a diluent, but as a therapeutic enhancer for bioactive plasma proteins, offering secondary benefits even though it reduces the per mL platelet concentration (Table 4.2).

## 4.5 Ultrafiltration of Plasma Proteins in Regenerative Medicine (Fig. 4.6)

Ultrafiltration is an advanced technique used to selectively concentrate regenerative plasma proteins by filtering based on their individual molecular weight. This is particularly valuable to enhance the therapeutic potency in pain management and orthopedic practices.

The process helps to recover regenerative proteins from plasma in clinically relevant volumes by using membrane filters with different pore sizes. This process preserves beneficial proteins like growth factors and cytokine inhibitors while allowing unwanted smaller molecules or debris to pass through. Figure 4.6 shows the different protein sizes and their ultrafiltration threshold.

*Ultrafiltration allows*:

Customization of plasma therapy based on protein targets
Enrichment of anti-inflammatory and anabolic mediators

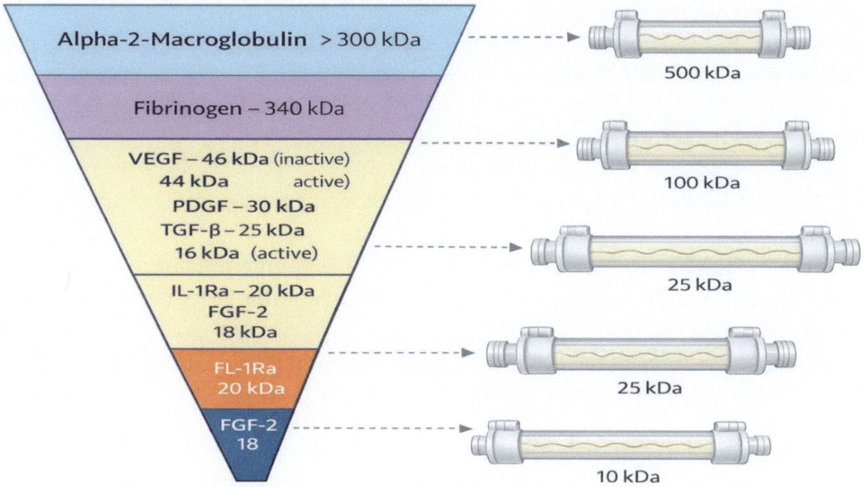


**Fig. 4.6** Ultrafiltration of plasma

Reduction in pro-inflammatory or excessive clotting proteins
Targeting inflammatory arthritis (e.g., enrich A2M, IRAP)
Promoting tissue repair (e.g., retain TGF-β, PDGF)
Avoiding unnecessary fibrinogen or large coagulation proteins

### 4.5.1 Alpha-2-Macroglobulin (A2M) and Its Therapeutic Utility

Alpha-2-macroglobulin (A2M) is a large plasma protein produced primarily by the liver and present in blood plasma. It acts as a broad-spectrum protease inhibitor, playing a critical role in tissue homeostasis, inflammation control, and joint preservation.

#### 4.5.1.1 Mechanism of Action

A2M functions by trapping and inactivating a wide variety of proteases, including those responsible for the degradation of extracellular matrix (ECM) components, such as matrix metalloproteinases (MMPs) and other inflammatory enzymes. These enzymes are often upregulated in conditions like osteoarthritis and contribute significantly to the breakdown of articular cartilage surfaces.

By inhibiting these proteases, A2M slows the progression of arthritis and joint degeneration.

The protein forms a complex with the proteases, rendering them inactive and facilitating their clearance from the body.

**Anti-Inflammatory Properties**
In addition to its protease inhibition, A2M also binds to and neutralizes pro-inflammatory cytokines such as:

Tumor necrosis factor-alpha (TNF-α)
Transforming growth factor-beta (TGF-β)
Interleukin-1 beta (IL-1β)

These cytokines are heavily implicated in chronic inflammatory responses and joint degradation. By neutralizing them the inflammation is reduced, resulting in less pain for patients.

Cellular repair mechanisms are facilitated, allowing local cells within the joint to engage in regeneration of the extracellular matrix (ECM).

#### 4.5.1.2 Clinical Application

In a regenerative setting, A2M is concentrated from platelet-poor plasma (PPP) derived from either peripheral blood or bone marrow aspirate (BMA). For example:

From 60 mL of whole blood, approximately 30 mL of PPP can be isolated.
This is further processed to yield 3–5 mL of concentrated A2M-rich plasma, which can then be injected into the affected joint or tissue.
This treatment offers a minimally invasive, biologically based option for managing arthritis and degenerative joint disease without the systemic effects of pharmacological therapies.

### 4.5.2 Interleukin-1 Receptor Antagonist Protein (IRAP)—Precision Blocking of Inflammation

IRAP, or interleukin-1 receptor antagonist protein, represents a specific and potent tool in regenerative medicine focused on cytokine modulation, particularly aimed at interleukin-1 (IL-1), a key driver of inflammation in joint and musculoskeletal diseases.

#### 4.5.2.1 Mechanism of Action

IL-1 is a pro-inflammatory cytokine that binds to IL-1 receptors (IL-1RI) on various cell types including the following:

Macrophages, monocytes, and osteoclasts
This interaction initiates a cascade of signaling events that promote inflammation, tissue degradation, and pain.

IRAP works by:

Blocking IL-1 receptors, effectively preventing IL-1 from binding and triggering downstream inflammatory signaling.

This reduces pain and slows down the degradation of both bone and cartilage matrix, especially in chronic degenerative conditions such as osteoarthritis.

Broader Immunomodulatory Effects: of IRAP:

IRAP also indirectly reduces the activation of immune and inflammatory cells:

- It dampens macrophage activity, reducing the production of other inflammatory cytokines.
- It inhibits monocyte and osteoclast activation, leading to decreased bone resorption and joint damage.

#### 4.5.2.2 Clinical Insights

IRAP is extracted and concentrated from platelet-poor plasma. Its efficacy is greatly enhanced when derived from bone marrow aspirate (BMA). In fact, IRAP levels in BMA plasma can be 11 to 22 times greater than in peripheral blood plasma.

This makes BMA a superior source for IRAP when preparing autologous biologics for injection.

This targeted approach enables precise modulation of specific cytokine pathways, offering a tailored therapy for inflammatory joint disease without the broad immunosuppressive effects of traditional drugs.

## 4.6 Summary (Table 4.3)

Both A2M and IRAP represent significant advancements in the field of biologic and regenerative pain medicine, providing effective, biologically targeted, and minimally invasive alternatives for managing chronic joint and musculoskeletal conditions (Table 4.3).

**Table 4.3** Summary

| Therapeutic agent | Key action | Biological effects | Clinical relevance |
|---|---|---|---|
| A2M | Inhibits proteases and pro-inflammatory cytokines (e.g., TNF-α, IL-1β) | Reduces cartilage breakdown and inflammation, promotes ECM repair | Used in arthritis to slow disease progression |
| IRAP | Blocks IL-1 receptor | Reduces inflammation and bone/cartilage destruction | Effective for joint pain, particularly from IL-1 driven inflammation |

### 4.6.1 Role of Extended PRP with PPP in the Pro-inflammatory Environment of Arthritis and Degenerative Conditions

PRP therapy has emerged as a biologic intervention capable of modulating the course of joint degeneration, particularly in the early to moderate stages of osteoarthritis. The pathological environment of degenerative joint and musculoskeletal diseases is marked by the persistent presence of pro-inflammatory mediators, which promote tissue degradation, pain, and impaired healing.

#### 4.6.1.1 Mechanism of Action of PRP

Platelet-rich plasma is derived from a patient's own blood and contains a high concentration of platelets, which are rich in growth factors such as:

Platelet-derived growth factor (PDGF)
Transforming growth factor-beta (TGF-β)
Insulin-like growth factor-1 (IGF-1)
Vascular endothelial growth factor (VEGF)

Cytokines and bioactive proteins reduce inflammation and stimulate tissue repair. The inflammatory protein mediators include the following:

Interleukin-1 beta (IL-1β): A master cytokine that drives inflammation and cartilage catabolism
Tumor necrosis factor-alpha (TNF-α): Enhances inflammation and synergizes with IL-1β
Matrix metalloproteinases (MMPs): Enzymes that degrade extracellular matrix and cartilage

These molecules create a hostile biochemical milieu that impedes regeneration and contributes to disease progression.

#### 4.6.1.2 Anti-Inflammatory and Anabolic Role of PRP

PRP is rich in bioactive molecules capable of modulating a hostile environment. Upon activation, platelets release a host of cytokines and many growth factors, including:

*Anabolic factors*:

Platelet-derived growth factor (PDGF)
Insulin-like growth factor-1 (IGF-1)
Transforming growth factor-beta (TGF-β)

These promote cell proliferation, tissue remodeling, and extracellular matrix production.

*Anti-inflammatory proteins*:

- Interleukin-1 Receptor Antagonist Protein (IRAP): Blocks IL-1β receptor signaling
- Alpha-2-Macroglobulin (A2M): Neutralizes proteases and inflammatory cytokines

Together, these factors offer potent, prolonged anti-inflammatory effects that counterbalance degenerative processes.

*When PRP is injected into joints, it has following effects*:

- PRP reduces inflammation, thereby decreasing the activity of cartilage-damaging enzymes.
- It stimulates the activity of chondrocytes (cartilage-producing cells) and promotes extracellular matrix synthesis.
- It enhances the quality of synovial fluid, improving joint lubrication and overall joint function.
- PRP also has an analgesic effect, which may be partially mediated by 5-hydroxytryptamine (5-HT or serotonin) release. Once platelets are activated, they release 5-HT from their storage in dense granules, thereby contributing to nociceptive modulation and pain relief.

### 4.6.2 Understanding Cartilage Degeneration and the Protective Role of PRP

#### 4.6.2.1 Natural Cartilage Loss Over Time

Articular cartilage is the smooth, white tissue that covers the ends of bones in joints. It allows bones to glide over each other with minimal friction, facilitating smooth and pain-free movement. However, cartilage has a limited capacity to heal because it is avascular (lacking blood supply), and its regenerative potential naturally declines with age.

Scientific observations suggest that humans lose approximately 5% of their cartilage volume per year, particularly in weight-bearing joints such as the knees and hips.

This loss is often asymptomatic in early stages but can gradually lead to joint stiffness, reduced range of motion, and eventually osteoarthritis (OA).

The rate of degeneration can be accelerated by factors such as aging, obesity, repetitive joint stress, injury, or inflammation.

This degenerative process, if left unchecked, leads to:

Progressive joint damage
Chronic pain and disability
The eventual need for joint replacement surgery

#### 4.6.2.2 Clinical Evidence

Studies and clinical trials have shown that PRP can reduce or halt the progression of osteoarthritis in up to 73% of cases, particularly when administered early in the disease course. Patients receiving PRP treatments report:

- Reduced pain
- Improved joint mobility
- Better quality of life

Imaging studies have also shown slower cartilage thinning and reduced joint space narrowing in patients treated with PRP compared to controls.

This makes PRP one of the most promising autologous (self-derived) regenerative therapies in modern musculoskeletal medicine.

While cartilage degeneration is a natural part of aging, regenerative interventions like PRP have shown promising results in altering the natural course of osteoarthritis. By leveraging the body's own healing components, PRP offers a minimally invasive, safe, and effective means to preserve joint integrity, reduce symptoms, and improve long-term outcomes for patients facing cartilage loss.

## 4.7 Important Regenerative Growth factors in PRP (Table 4.4)

**Table 4.4** Important regenerative growth factors in PRP

| Growth factor | Function |
|---|---|
| PDGF (platelet-derived growth factor) | Stimulates cell proliferation, chemotaxis, differentiation; promotes angiogenesis |
| TGF-β (transforming growth factor-beta) | Stimulates production of collagen type I & III, angiogenesis, re-epithelialization, inhibits collagen breakdown via protease inhibitors |
| VEGF (vascular endothelial growth factor) | Stimulates angiogenesis by regulating endothelial cell proliferation and migration |
| EGF (epidermal growth factor) | Promotes cell proliferation and cytoprotection, accelerates re-epithelialization, increases tensile strength, supports granulation tissue organization |
| bFGF (basic fibroblast growth factor) | Stimulates angiogenesis, promotes stem cell proliferation and collagen-based tissue repair |
| IGF-1 (insulin-like growth factor 1) | Regulates cell proliferation and differentiation, influences osteoblast matrix secretion and production of proteoglycans and collagen |

## 4.8 Clinical Applications of PRP in Musculoskeletal Pain

### 4.8.1 Efficacy of PRP in Knee Osteoarthritis

PRP is supported by multiple meta-analyses and guidelines, including those from the American Society of Pain and Neuroscience, as an effective therapy for knee osteoarthritis, providing clinically significant improvements in pain and function compared to placebo and hyaluronic acid, particularly with high-platelet concentration preparations. Benefits are most pronounced mild to moderate disease and can persist for up to 12 months. However, some high-quality trials, such as RESTORE RCT, have reported no significant difference between PRP and placebo, highlighting variability in outcomes likely related to differences in PRP formulation and study design.

### 4.8.2 Efficacy of PRP in Tendinopathies

PRP demonstrates variable efficacy across tendinopathies. There is strong evidence for benefit in lateral epicondylitis and some support for use in rotator cuff and plantar fasciopathy, particularly with leukocyte-rich PRP formulations. In contrast, high-quality meta-analyses indicate no clinically meaningful benefit for Achilles tendinopathy, and results for patellar tendinopathy are mixed. Efficacy appears to depend on tendon type, chronicity, and PRP characteristics.

### 4.8.3 Efficacy of PRP for Epidural Use in Radiculopathy Due to Disc Herniation

For lumbar radiculopathy secondary to disc herniation, meta-analyses and randomized trials show that epidural PRP provides pain and functional improvement comparable to epidural steroid injection (ESI), with a similar safety profile and possibly more durable benefit beyond 3–6 months. No increase in adverse events has been observed, and PRP is considered a viable alternative to steroids in this context.

### 4.8.4 Efficacy and Safety of PRP for Peripheral Neuropathy

Patients with diabetic peripheral neuropathy have demonstrated the most benefit from platelet-rich plasma (PRP) treatment among the peripheral neuropathic populations, based on the current evidence. Randomized controlled trials and systematic reviews consistently show that perineural PRP injections in diabetic peripheral neuropathy result in significant improvements in pain, numbness, and nerve function scores compared to standard medical therapy, with benefits persisting for up to 6 months. Treatment has a high safety profile. The American Society of Pain and

Neuroscience, in its 2024 guideline, specifically highlights PRP as an effective alternative approach for painful diabetic neuropathy, citing high-level evidence for pain and symptom reduction.

## 4.9 In Summary

Platelet-rich plasma is a promising and widely used orthobiologic with the most robust evidence in knee osteoarthritis and select tendinopathies.

Its use in peripheral neuropathy is safe and shows some promise.

PRP is considered safe and legal according to its FDA regulation status.

PRP is classified as minimally manipulated autologous tissue under FDA 361 HCT/P regulation, allowing off label use in musculoskeletal and pain management.

It is an autologous source which eliminates risk of immune rejection or disease transmission.

It has a safety profile as evidenced by extensive clinical experience which supports a low risk of infection, allergic reaction, or other complications.

There are some limitations and research gaps which include the following:

Lack of standardization: significant variability exists in PRP formulation, including platelet concentration, leukocyte content, and activation methods.

Outcome variability: differences in study design and patient selection contribute to inconsistent findings, particularly in tendinopathies and neuropathies.

Long-term data: while short- and medium-term efficacy is supported, high-quality long-term trials are needed to establish durability and optimal dosing protocols.

## Suggested Readings

American Medical Society for Sports Medicine (AMSSM). Position statement: orthobiologics in sports medicine. 2022. Retrieved from 2022. https://www.amssm.org

American Society of Pain and Neuroscience (ASPN). STEP guidelines: interventional treatments for knee pain and peripheral neuropathy. 2024. Retrieved from 2024. https://www.painneurosociety.com.

Andia I, Maffulli N. Platelet-rich plasma for managing pain and inflammation in osteoarthritis. Nat Rev Rheumatol. 2013;9(12):721–30.

Barreto A, et al. Alpha-2-macroglobulin in musculoskeletal medicine: a narrative review. Orthop J Sports Med. 2020;8(5):2325967120917063.

Belk JW, Kraeutler MJ, Houck DA, Goodrich LR, Dragoo JL, McCarty EC. Platelet-rich plasma versus hyaluronic acid for knee osteoarthritis: a systematic review and meta-analysis of randomized controlled trials. Am J Sports Med. 2021;49(1):249–60. https://doi.org/10.1177/0363546520909397.

Boswell SG, Cole BJ, Sundman EA, et al. Platelet-rich plasma: a milieu of bioactive factors. Arthroscopy. 2012;28(3):429–39.

Choudhury ME, Inoue T, Fukuda S. Platelet-rich plasma in peripheral neuropathy: a systematic review of current evidence. J Clin Med. 2021;10(11):2326. https://doi.org/10.3390/jcm10112326.

Degen RM, Bernard JA, Oliver KS, Dines JS. Commercial separation systems designed for preparation of platelet-rich plasma yield differences in cellular composition. HSS J. 2017;13(1):75–80. https://doi.org/10.1007/s11420-016-9517-4.

Dragoo JL, Braun HJ, Durham JL, et al. Comparison of the acute inflammatory response of two commercial platelet-rich plasma systems in healthy rabbit tendons. Am J Sports Med. 2012;40(6):1274–81.

Eckstein F, et al. Quantitative imaging of cartilage and bone morphology in osteoarthritis. Radiol Clin North Am. 2009;47(4):655–73.

Evans CH, Chevalier X, Wehling P. Autologous conditioned serum. Phys Med Rehabil Clin N Am. 2016;27(4):893–908.

Filardo G, et al. Platelet-rich plasma intra-articular knee injections for the treatment of degenerative cartilage lesions and osteoarthritis. Knee Surg Sports Traumatol Arthrosc. 2011;19(4):528–35.

Fitzpatrick J, Bulsara M, Zheng MH. The effectiveness of platelet-rich plasma in the treatment of tendinopathy: a meta-analysis of randomized controlled clinical trials. Am J Sports Med. 2017;45(1):226–33. https://doi.org/10.1177/0363546516637176.

Giusti I, et al. The optimal concentration of platelets for platelet-rich plasma: anti- and pro-angiogenic effects. J Cell Physiol. 2009;219(3):685–91.

Hunter DJ, et al. Structural correlates of pain in joints with osteoarthritis. Osteoarthr Cartil. 2013;21(9):1170–8.

Laudy ABM, et al. Efficacy of platelet-rich plasma injections in osteoarthritis of the knee: a systematic review and meta-analysis. Br J Sports Med. 2015;49(10):657–72.

Marx RE. Platelet-rich plasma: evidence to support its use. J Oral Maxillofac Surg. 2004;62(4):489–96.

McCarrel TM, Fortier LA. Temporal growth factor release from platelet-rich plasma, trehalose lyophilized platelets, and bone marrow aspirate and their effect on tendon and ligament gene expression. Am J Sports Med. 2009;37(6):1043–9.

Meheux CJ, et al. Efficacy of intra-articular platelet-rich plasma injections in knee osteoarthritis: a systematic review. Arthroscopy. 2016;32(3):495–505.

Mishra AK, Skrepnik NV, Edwards SG, et al. Efficacy of platelet-rich plasma for chronic tennis elbow: a double-blind, prospective, multicenter, randomized controlled trial of 230 patients. Am J Sports Med. 2014;42(2):463–71. https://doi.org/10.1177/0363546513518416.

Patel S, et al. Treatment with platelet-rich plasma is more effective than placebo for knee osteoarthritis: a prospective, double-blind, randomized trial. Am J Sports Med. 2013;41(2):356–64.

Sharma L, et al. The role of biomechanics and inflammation in osteoarthritis. Arthritis Rheum. 2006;54(5):1580–6.

Shen L, Yuan T, Chen S, Xie X, Zhang C, Lei G. The temporal effect of platelet-rich plasma on pain and physical function in the treatment of knee osteoarthritis: systematic review and meta-analysis of randomized controlled trials. J Orthop Surg Res. 2017;12:16. https://doi.org/10.1186/s13018-017-0521-5.

Textor JA, Tablin F. Inflammatory cell gene expression in response to platelet-rich plasma in horses. Vet Immunol Immunopathol. 2013;155(1–2):27–36.

Tuakli-Wosornu YA, Terry A, Boachie-Adjei K, Harrison J, Riew KD. Epidural platelet-rich plasma injection for lumbar radiculopathy: a preliminary report. Pain Med. 2016;17(10):1814–24. https://doi.org/10.1093/pm/pnv088.

Wu YT, Ho TY, Chou LW, Ke MJ, Li TY, Tsai CK. Effectiveness of platelet-rich plasma injections in patients with diabetic peripheral neuropathy: a randomized controlled trial. J Tissue Eng Regen Med. 2018;12(6):e1186–92. https://doi.org/10.1002/term.2625.

# Mesenchymal Stem Cells

5

Ripu D. Arora and Sheri L. Albers

## 5.1 What Is a Stem Cell?

A mesenchymal stem cell (MSC) is a type of primitive, undifferentiated cell with remarkable potential to transform and heal. Although they are fairly ubiquitous, these cells are primarily derived from bone marrow, fat tissue, and umbilical cord sources. MSCs play a pivotal role in tissue repair and immune modulation through their secretion of trophic or signaling factors. Because they do not solely behave as tissue progenitors in the body, as Dr. Arnold Caplan proposed, a better term for them is Medicinal Signaling Cells.

*Mesenchymal stem cells (MSCs) possess the following abilities*:

1. Self-Replication
   Stem cells can self-replicate, meaning they divide and produce identical daughter cells. This intrinsic ability ensures a sustained pool of stem cells that can be mobilized for tissue repair and immune regulation throughout the lifespan of the individual.
2. Differentiation into Multiple Tissues
   MSC's most significant feature is their multipotency which means they possess the ability to differentiate into various cell lineages derived from the three germ layers:
   *Ectoderm*: Neurons, epithelial cells
   *Endoderm*: Muscle cells, gut epithelial cells, lung cells
   *Mesoderm*: Osteocytes, chondrocytes, adipocytes, endothelial cells, and myocytes

R. D. Arora (✉)
Arora Pain Clinic, Torrance, CA, USA

S. L. Albers
Radiology Research and Consultation, Sacramento, CA, USA

 
R. D. Arora (ed.), *Regenerative Medicine in Pain Practice*,
https://doi.org/10.1007/978-3-032-22644-0_5

This ability enables them to replace damaged or diseased cells with regenerative therapies.

This allows targeted regeneration in orthopedic, musculoskeletal, and even some neurological applications.

3. Migration and Homing
MSCs can actively migrate to sites of tissue injury or inflammation through ligand-receptor interactions. This targeted migration is crucial for localized tissue repair, especially in systemic administration.
4. Paracrine Effect
Rather than solely depending on direct cell replacement, MSCs exert significant therapeutic benefits through the secretion of paracrine factors as well as trophic factors. These factors initiate and support tissue healing, angiogenesis, and regeneration by modulating the surrounding microenvironment.
5. Immunomodulatory Function
MSCs by direct contact and through secreted factors can modulate the immune response by reducing inflammation and suppressing immune cell activation. This property is especially beneficial in preventing transplant rejection and treating autoimmune conditions. The cells help in fighting infection and modify immunity.
6. Fight Apoptosis (Cell Death)
Stem cells can inhibit apoptosis, the process of programmed cell death. In degenerative conditions, surrounding tissues often undergo apoptosis due to inflammation or trauma. MSCs help protect these tissues, promote survival, and support regeneration.
7. Reduce Inflammation
One of the most clinically valuable properties of MSCs is their ability to modulate the immune system and suppress inflammation. By reducing inflammatory cytokines and promoting anti-inflammatory factors, stem cells help relieve chronic pain, particularly in joints, the spine, and soft tissues.

## 5.2 Understanding Stem Cell Potency and Its Clinical Implications

Stem cells are categorized based on their potency and the capacity to differentiate into different cell types. The hierarchy of stem cell potency includes totipotent, pluripotent, and multipotent stem cells, each of these have unique biological roles and therapeutic potential.

### 5.2.1 Totipotent Stem Cells

**Definition** Totipotent stem cells are the most versatile of all stem cell types. They can give rise to all cell types in an organism, including both embryonic (all body tissues) and extra-embryonic (placental) tissues.

These cells are derived from the fertilized egg (zygote) and are present during the first few divisions following fertilization.

While totipotent cells hold enormous regenerative potential, their application in clinical settings is limited due to ethical and technical challenges.

A single totipotent cell can develop into an entire organism, making it the starting point of human development.

### 5.2.2 Pluripotent Stem Cells

**Definition** Pluripotent stem cells can give rise to all cell types derived from the three germ layers, which are ectoderm, mesoderm, and endoderm. These include every tissue in the human body, but not the placenta.

These cells are isolated from the inner cell mass of the blastocyst, an early-stage embryo, e.g., embryonic stem cells (ESCs) and induced pluripotent stem cells (iPSCs).

Pluripotent cells offer potential in developing therapies for neurodegenerative conditions, spinal cord injuries, and other complex pain syndromes through neural and musculoskeletal tissue regeneration.

The use of ESCs involves destruction of the embryo, leading to ongoing ethical debates in research and clinical application.

### 5.2.3 Multipotent Stem Cells (Fig. 5.1)

Multipotent stem cells are limited in their differentiation potential. They can develop into a restricted range of cell types within a specific tissue or organ system.

They are found in adult tissues, such as bone marrow, fat, and umbilical cord blood, dermis, and synovium (Table 5.1).

**Different Types of Stem Cells (Fig. 5.2)**
Hematopoietic Stem Cells (HSCs): Differentiate into blood cells.
Mesenchymal Stem Cells (MSCs): Give rise to bone, cartilage, muscle, and fat.
Neural Stem Cells (NSCs): Develop into neurons and glial cells.

**Clinical Applications in Pain**
Osteoarthritis: MSCs used for cartilage repair.
Intervertebral Disc Degeneration: Stem cell injections promote disc regeneration.
Peripheral Neuropathy: NSCs explored for nerve regeneration.

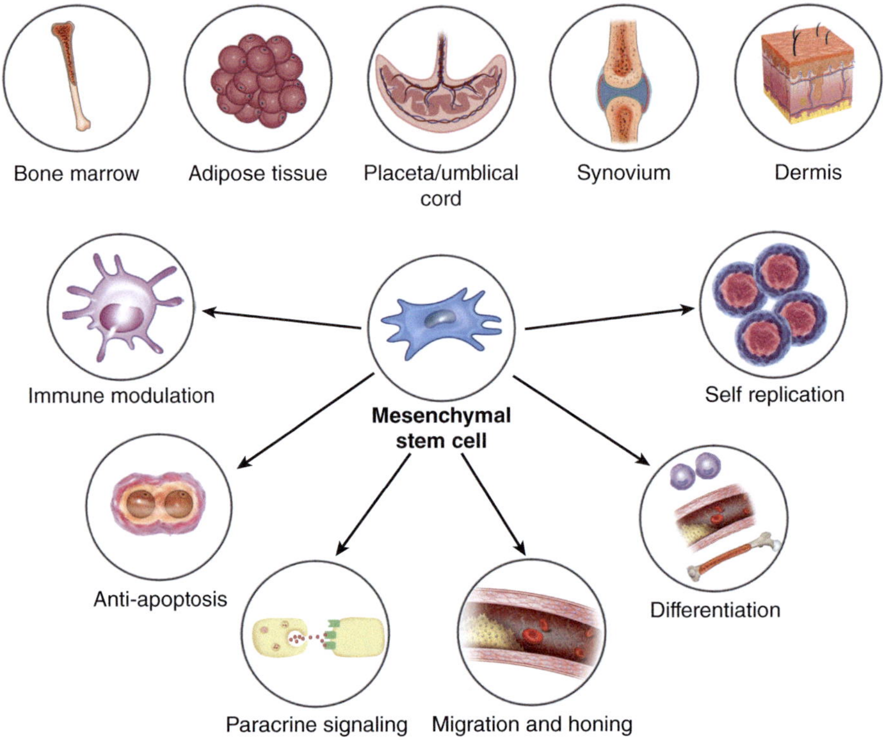


**Fig. 5.1** Mesenchymal stem cell and its functions. Mesenchymal stem cells (MSCs) are multipotent stromal cells capable of self-renewal and differentiation into a variety of cell types. They are isolated from multiple tissue sources, including bone marrow, adipose tissue, umbilical cord (including cord blood and placenta), dermis, synovial membrane, dental pulp, and periodontal ligaments

**Table 5.1** Summary of stem cell potency

| Stem cell type | Potency | Differentiates into | Source | Clinical use |
|---|---|---|---|---|
| Totipotent | Highest | All body and placental cells | Fertilized egg | No direct clinical use; research only |
| Pluripotent | High | All body cells (not placenta) | Embryo, iPSCs | High potential; limited by ethics |
| Multipotent | Moderate | Specific tissue lineages (e.g., MSCs) | Adult tissues | Widely used in pain and tissue therapies |

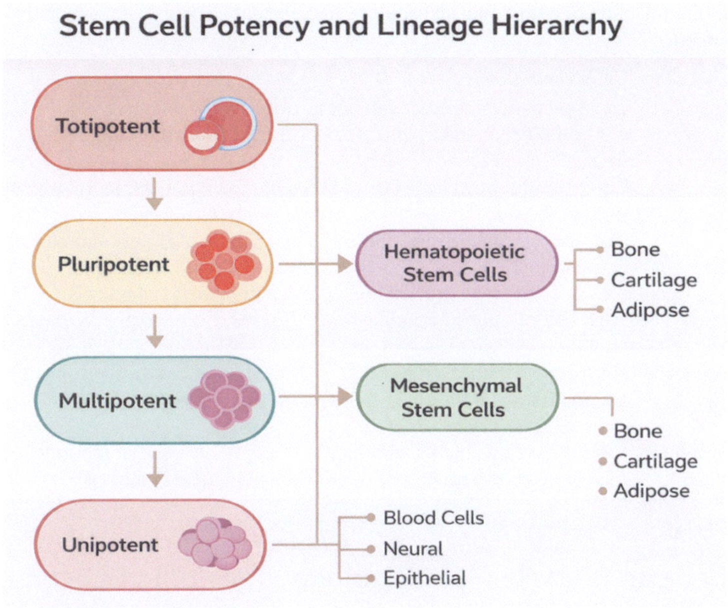


**Fig. 5.2** Different types of stem cells

## 5.3 Comparison of Embryonic and Adult Stem Cells in Regenerative Medicine

In the field of regenerative medicine and pain practice, stem cells are evaluated based on their origin, potency, safety, and clinical applicability. Two primary categories are ESCs and adult stem cells (ASCs), each with distinct characteristics (Table 5.2).

*ESCs* are totipotent, capable of differentiating into any cell type including placental tissues. They are easily harvested in large quantities but pose significant ethical concerns and a high risk of immune rejection and tumor formation (e.g., teratomas). As a result, their use remains largely experimental and is limited by legal and regulatory frameworks.

*In contrast*, ASCs especially MSCs derived from bone marrow or adipose tissue are multipotent and safer for clinical use. These cells are often used autologously, reducing the risk of immune response and ethical complications. Although they are harder to isolate and expand, they are widely used in musculoskeletal and degenerative conditions to reduce inflammation and promote tissue repair (Fig. 5.3).

In summary, ASCs are currently the preferred choice in clinical pain practice due to their safety profile, ethical acceptability, and established efficacy in conditions such as osteoarthritis, tendon injuries, and discogenic pain. ESCs hold great theoretical promise but are not yet viable for routine clinical use.

**Table 5.2** Comparison of embryonic and adult stem cells in the context of regenerative medicine and pain practice

| Feature | Embryonic stem cells | Adult stem cells |
|---|---|---|
| Potency | *Totipotent*—Can differentiate into any cell type, including placental tissues | *Multipotent or pluripotent*—Can differentiate into limited cell types |
| Source availability | Large numbers can be harvested from embryos | Limited numbers; more difficult to isolate from tissues |
| Immune response | May cause immune rejection since non-autologous | Less likely to cause immune rejection; patient's own cells can be used (autologous) |
| Tumor risk | High risk of tumor formation (e.g., teratomas) | Lower risk of tumor formation |
| Ethical and legal issues | High ethical controversy and uncertain legal status due to embryo use | Minimal ethical issues; legally accepted in most settings |
| Clinical use in pain practice | Limited due to ethical and tumor risks; mostly experimental | Commonly used in musculoskeletal and degenerative conditions |

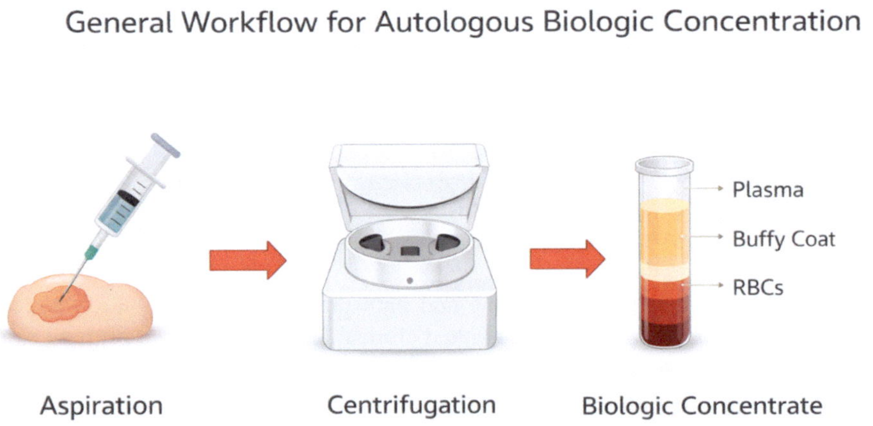


**Fig. 5.3** Formation of BMAC

## 5.4 MSCs from Bone Marrow Aspirate Creation

### 5.4.1 Bone Marrow Aspiration (Fig. 5.3)

**Site** Typically aspirated from the posterior iliac crest (pelvis).

**Technique**
A special needle is inserted into the spongy bone area (trabecular bone) rich in marrow.

A volume of bone marrow (usually 30–60 mL) is aspirated, using six 10 mL syringes for better concentration of MSCs.

**Content**
The aspirate contains a mixture of blood, HSCs, MSCs, plasma, and other stromal elements.

### 5.4.2 Concentration via Centrifugation

*Device*: Automated centrifuge
Purpose: To separate and concentrate the cellular components
Mechanism: Centrifugation uses density gradients to isolate cell layers:
Top Layer: Plasma
Middle Layer: Buffy coat which is rich in mononuclear cells, including MSCs
Bottom Layer: Red blood cells

### 5.4.3 Collection of MSC-Rich Layer

The buffy coat is carefully extracted. It contains MSCs which are multipotent stromal cells capable of differentiating into cartilage, bone, muscle, and fat. Platelets and growth factors are also found in this layer which aid in healing and tissue regeneration.

### 5.4.4 Advantages of Bone Marrow–Derived MSCs

Constitutes autologous use which minimizes immune rejection.

The procedure is minimally invasive and can be performed as an office-based or ambulatory care procedure.

Its regenerative capabilities make it especially valuable in orthopedics, sports medicine, and spine interventions.

### 5.4.5 Clinical Application

Injection into target areas for repair and regeneration such as joints (e.g., knees, shoulders), intervertebral discs, tendons, and ligaments.

**Clinical Goals**
Reduce inflammation
Promote tissue repair and regeneration
Improve function
Reduce chronic pain

## 5.5 Impact of Aging on Stem Cell Availability and Regenerative Potential

A critical factor in the effectiveness of regenerative therapies such as stem cell and platelet-rich plasma (PRP) injections is the availability and functional capacity of stem cells, which decline progressively with age. This age-related reduction directly influences healing potential, tissue regeneration, and clinical outcomes in pain and injury management.

With advancing age, stem cells become fewer in number and less efficient in their function, leading to a diminished regenerative capacity (Fig. 5.4). This decline contributes to slower repair of damaged tissues and a reduced response to biologic therapies. In contrast, younger sources, such as those derived from birth-associated tissues, contain stem cells with higher proliferation rates and stronger regenerative potential, making them especially advantageous for therapeutic use.

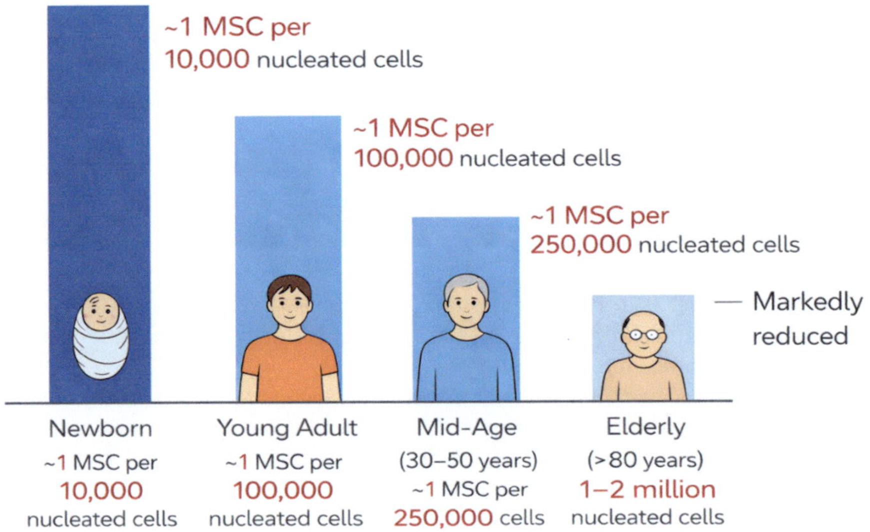


**Fig. 5.4** Age-related decline in bone marrow mesenchymal stem cell (MSC) frequency. The frequency of mesenchymal stem cells within the bone marrow decreases progressively with age. In newborns, MSCs are present at an approximate frequency of 1 per 10,000 nucleated cells. This declines to approximately 1 per 100,000 cells in young adults, further decreases to around 1 per 250,000 cells in mid-life, and reaches approximately 1 per 1–2 million nucleated cells in elderly individuals. The illustration depicts relative age-associated trends rather than absolute quantitative measurements

## 5.6 Clinical Relevance in Pain Medicine

Musculoskeletal pain and degenerative conditions often involve tissues such as cartilage, tendons, and intervertebral discs which naturally possess limited self-repair capacity. This limitation is magnified with age, as the pool of resident stem and progenitor cells declines in both number and function. As a result, older tissues struggle to mount an effective regenerative response after injury or wear.

For the practicing clinician, patient age and stem cell quality must be considered when selecting and tailoring regenerative treatment protocols. Reduced performance of autologous cells in older individuals has led to increased interest in allogeneic stem cell sources from younger donors. Perinatal tissues such as umbilical cord blood are particularly attractive, as they contain stem cells with superior proliferative ability, higher regenerative potential, and greater capacity to support tissue repair. This rationale explains why younger donor-derived sources are frequently explored as therapeutic options for aging patients.

The progressive decline in stem cell concentration and function represents a fundamental barrier in regenerative medicine. For effective pain management in older populations, strategies must evolve to address this biological limitation. Potential solutions include the following:

- Utilizing younger donor-derived cell sources with enhanced regenerative potential
- Optimizing harvest sites in autologous procedures to maximize viable cell yield
- Employing cell-preserving and enhancing technologies to maintain stem cell viability and functionality

By integrating these approaches, clinicians can better overcome age-related constraints and achieve more consistent outcomes in the management of pain and degenerative musculoskeletal conditions.

## 5.7 Clinical Applications in Pain Practice

MSCs play a pivotal role in regenerative medicine due to their multipotential differentiation capacity, immunomodulatory functions, and paracrine signaling. They can differentiate into bone, cartilage, muscle, tendon, and fat cells and are commonly sourced from bone marrow, adipose tissue, periosteum, and other mesenchymal tissues. Their regenerative and anti-inflammatory properties have been investigated across a spectrum of musculoskeletal conditions, including osteoarthritis, ligament and tendon injuries, meniscal tears, muscle damage, and intervertebral disc degeneration.

Stem cell therapy is emerging as a promising non-surgical alternative in many musculoskeletal conditions such as osteoarthritis (e.g., knee, hip, shoulder), tendon and ligament Injuries, spinal disc degeneration, post-surgical pain, and in

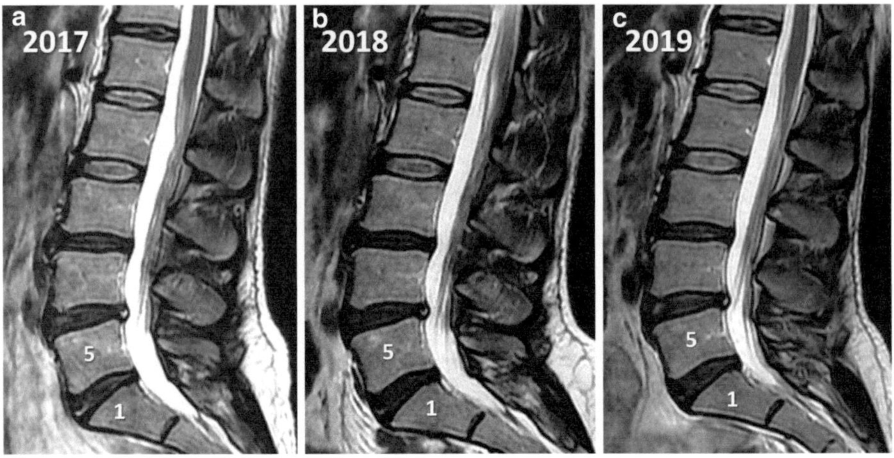


**Fig. 5.5** Serial sagittal T2-weighted MRI of the lumbar spine following intradiscal bone marrow aspirate concentrate (BMAC) injection. (**a**) Sagittal T2-weighted MRI demonstrates multilevel degenerative disc disease involving L3–L4, L4–L5, and L5–S1. The L5–S1 disc, which was clinically symptomatic, shows reduced disc height and an anterior annular fissure. (**b**) Follow-up sagittal T2-weighted MRI obtained approximately 1 year after intradiscal BMAC injection at L5–S1 demonstrates a mild interval increase in disc height, with decreased conspicuity of the anterior annular fissure. The patient reported interval improvement in low back pain. (**c**) Follow-up sagittal T2-weighted MRI obtained approximately 2 years after intradiscal BMAC injection demonstrates a further mild increase in L5–S1 disc height, with the anterior annular fissure now minimally perceptible. The patient reported sustained clinical improvement with improved functional status

neuropathic pain. With ongoing research, MSC-based treatments continue to expand into broader areas of chronic pain and tissue degeneration (Fig. 5.5).

In osteoarthritis, intra-articular MSC therapy has shown promise in reducing pain, improving joint function, and supporting cartilage regeneration, accompanied by supporting evidence from imaging and arthroscopy. Both bone marrow–derived and adipose-derived MSCs appear to offer comparable clinical outcomes.

For tendon and ligament injuries, MSCs contribute through tenogenic differentiation, secretion of growth factors, and enhancement of local vascularization and extracellular matrix remodeling.

In bone healing, MSCs support osteogenesis and modulate the microenvironment to accelerate repair. MSCs also support angiogenesis, and with their paracrine effects, enhance the local regenerative milieu.

## 5.8 MSC-Derived Extracellular Vehicles (EVs)

A growing area of interest is the use of MSC-derived exosomes and extracellular vehicles (EVs). These vesicles deliver bioactive molecules such as microRNAs, proteins, and cytokines, which mediate many of the regenerative and immunomodulatory effects of MSCs. They represent a cell-free therapeutic alternative with low immunogenic and tumorigenic risks.

### 5.8.1 Safety and Cancer Considerations

While early clinical studies support the safety of MSC-based and MSC-derived EV therapies, long-term data are still limited. The relationship between stem cell therapies and cancer risk remains complex. Preclinical studies show that MSC-derived EVs can exert both pro-tumorigenic and anti-tumorigenic effects, depending on their molecular content, source tissue, and host environment. This is particularly relevant in patients with metabolic comorbidities like obesity, type 2 diabetes, and cardiovascular disease, where chronic inflammation may influence the biological response to therapy. However, to date, no clinical studies have shown an increased cancer risk or recurrence in patients treated with MSC-EV therapies for musculoskeletal disorders.

There are no universally accepted, specific absolute contraindications for the use of MSCs in the treatment of musculoskeletal disorders such as knee osteoarthritis, tendon and ligament injuries, meniscal tears, muscle injuries, and degenerative disc disease. The current clinical literature and guidelines, including those from the American Society of Pain and Neuroscience, consistently report that MSC therapy is generally safe, with most adverse events being mild and self-limited (e.g., joint pain, swelling, injection site pain, effusion). Severe adverse events are rare but have been reported (e.g., dyslipidemia, anemia, muscle hemorrhage, severe bursitis), all of which resolved without long-term sequelae.

## 5.9 Clinical Evidence for Mesenchymal Stem Cell Therapy in Musculoskeletal Disorders

Mesenchymal stem cell (MSC) therapy is a rapidly evolving treatment modality in regenerative medicine, particularly for knee osteoarthritis (OA) which is the most well-studied and prevalent musculoskeletal condition responsive to stem cell interventions. According to a 2023 publication in the *European Journal of Medical Research*, a growing body of randomized controlled trials and systematic reviews demonstrates that intra-articular MSC injections improve pain and functional outcomes in knee OA. Imaging modalities such as MRI and arthroscopy have shown evidence of cartilage regeneration, although the long-term durability and extent of structural repair remain areas of active investigation.

The American Society of Pain and Neuroscience (ASPN), through its STEP Guidelines, supports the use of autologous MSCs from either bone marrow or adipose tissue in knee OA, noting comparable efficacy across sources for symptom relief and functional improvement.

For other musculoskeletal conditions such as tendon and ligament injuries, meniscal tears, muscle injuries, and degenerative disc disease, early clinical studies and case series have reported improved healing and functional outcomes. However, these applications remain investigational, with limited high-quality, large-scale clinical trial data to support routine clinical use.

## 5.10 Clinical Evidence Supporting Bone Marrow Aspirate Concentrate (BMAC) in Cartilage Repair

BMAC has emerged as one of the most biologically potent and clinically effective autologous cell-based therapies for cartilage injuries and osteoarthritis. BMAC provides a concentrated population of mesenchymal stem/stromal cells (MSCs), hematopoietic progenitors, platelets, and growth factors that collectively promote inflammation modulation, matrix remodeling, angiogenesis, and tissue regeneration.

### 5.10.1 Study 1—Clinical Improvement Following BMAC Injection

Short-term clinical efficacy of BMAC has been demonstrated in patients with knee osteoarthritis. In a prospective clinical study, Subramanyam et al. evaluated intra-articular BMAC injections and reported significant reductions in pain and improvements in functional outcomes including visual analog scale (VAS), Knee Injury and Osteoarthritis Outcome Score (KOOS), and WOMAC scores at 6-month follow-up. These improvements were achieved with a single BMAC injection and without serious adverse events, confirming both the safety and short-term therapeutic efficacy of BMAC in degenerative joint disease [1].

### 5.10.2 Study 2—Systematic Review and Meta-Analytic Evidence

The growing clinical use of BMAC is supported by systematic reviews of orthobiologics therapies. Keeling et al. conducted a systematic review of bone marrow aspirate concentrate for knee osteoarthritis and concluded that intra-articular BMAC produces consistent improvements in pain and function across multiple clinical studies [2]. These findings confirm that autologous cell-based therapies provide clinically meaningful benefit in osteoarthritic joints and support the inclusion of BMAC in regenerative pain management algorithms.

### 5.10.3 Study 3—Structural Cartilage Regeneration with BMAC

Beyond symptomatic improvement, BMAC has demonstrated the capacity to promote true cartilage regeneration when combined with biological scaffolds.

Gobbi et al. reported a 24-month observational study of BMAC-augmented cartilage repair in 15 patients, demonstrating complete defect filling on MRI in approximately 80% of cases. Histologic analysis confirmed the presence of hyaline-like cartilage, indicating true tissue regeneration rather than fibrocartilaginous repair [3].

In a subsequent prospective study, Gobbi et al. followed 25 patients with full-thickness chondral defects for a mean of 41 months and observed significant improvements in KOOS, IKDC, Lysholm, Marx, and Tegner scores. MRI again demonstrated complete defect filling in 80% of patients, with superior outcomes observed in younger patients and those with isolated lesions [4].

Similarly, Enea et al. combined BMAC with microfracture and a collagen scaffold and demonstrated significant improvements in IKDC, Lysholm, and VAS scores, with second-look arthroscopy and histologic analysis confirming regeneration of hyaline-like cartilage [5].

These studies establish that BMAC provides both clinical improvement and biologically meaningful structural cartilage restoration.

### 5.10.4 Study 4—Comparative Evidence: BMAC Versus PRP

Direct comparative evidence further supports the regenerative superiority of BMAC. El-Kadiry et al. compared intra-articular BMAC with PRP in patients with knee osteoarthritis over 12 months. The BMAC group demonstrated significantly greater reductions in pain and superior functional improvement compared with PRP. MRI analysis revealed higher-quality cartilage repair in the BMAC group, indicating enhanced biological and structural regeneration [6].

These findings confirm that BMAC offers advantages over PRP not only in symptom relief but also in restoration of hyaline-like cartilage.

## 5.11 Conclusion

The collective evidence from these studies highlights the clinical expectancy of BMAC as a regenerative biologic in the treatment of cartilage damage. Improvements in functional scores, promising radiologic findings, and histological evidence of hyaline-like cartilage formation support its application across a range of orthopedic and pain management settings. Patient selection, particularly age and lesion characteristics, remains critical to optimizing outcomes. As evidence accumulates, BMAC is poised to become an integral component of biologically driven cartilage repair strategies. The future of regenerative pain therapy will likely integrate cell-based and cell-free (EVs) therapeutic advances in molecular profiling and individualized treatment planning.

## 5.12 Comparison of PRP and Stem Cell Therapy in Pain Practice

| Criteria | Platelet-rich plasma (PRP) | Stem cell therapy |
|---|---|---|
| Regeneration potential | Stimulates natural healing but does not regenerate lost tissues | Can differentiate into various cell types and regenerate damaged tissues |
| Efficacy in advanced cases | Limited in severe degenerative conditions | More effective for advanced and chronic degenerative conditions |
| Procedure complexity | Simple outpatient procedure (blood draw, centrifuge, and injection) | Requires specialized harvesting, processing, and injection techniques |
| Cost and availability | More affordable and widely available | More expensive and requires advanced lab processing |
| Condition | Mild/moderate indications | Advanced/severe indications |
| Joint and cartilage disorders | Mild to moderate osteoarthritis (e.g., knees, shoulders, hips, ankles) | Advanced osteoarthritis, cartilage defects, and avascular necrosis |
| Tendon and ligament injuries | Medial and lateral epicondylitis, Achilles tendinopathy, rotator cuff tendinopathy, patellar tendonitis | Severe tendon or ligament injuries, partial tears, and chronic tendon degeneration |
| Spine and disc issues | Mild disc degeneration, facet joint syndrome | Degenerative disc disease, spinal cord injuries, and chronic back pain |
| Muscle injuries | Muscle strains and mild tears | Severe muscle injuries, fibrosis, and atrophic conditions |
| Wound healing and skin rejuvenation | Diabetic ulcers, skin burns, hair loss (alopecia) | Non-healing wounds, extensive tissue damage, and reconstructive applications |
| Autoimmune and inflammatory conditions | Mild inflammatory arthritis | Rheumatoid arthritis, multiple sclerosis, lupus (research ongoing) |
| Regeneration potential | Stimulates natural healing but does not regenerate lost tissues | Can differentiate into various cell types and regenerate damaged tissues |
| Efficacy in advanced cases | Limited in severe degenerative conditions | More effective for advanced and chronic degenerative conditions |
| Procedure complexity | Simple outpatient procedure (blood draw, centrifuge, and injection) | Requires specialized harvesting, processing, and injection techniques |
| Cost and availability | More affordable and widely available | More expensive and requires advanced lab processing |

## References

1. Subramanyam K, Poornima S, Kumar S, Hasan Q. Short-term clinical results of single-injection autologous bone marrow aspirate concentrate in knee osteoarthritis. Biologics. 2024;4(2):218–31.
2. Keeling LE, Belk JW, Kraeutler MJ, McCarty EC, Postma WF. Bone marrow aspirate concentrate for the treatment of knee osteoarthritis: a systematic review. Am J Sports Med. 2022;50(9):2315–23.

3. Gobbi A, Karnatzikos G, Scotti C, et al. One-step cartilage repair with bone marrow aspirate concentrate and hyaluronic acid scaffold. Knee Surg Sports Traumatol Arthrosc. 2011;2(3):286–99. https://doi.org/10.1177/1947603510392023.
4. Gobbi A, Whyte GP. Long-term outcomes of bone marrow aspirate concentrate-based cartilage repair. Am J Sports Med. 2019;47(7):1621–8. https://doi.org/10.1177/0363546519845362. Epub 2019 May 16.
5. Enea D, Cecconi S, Calcagno S, et al. Single-stage cartilage repair with bone marrow aspirate concentrate and collagen membrane. Knee Surg Sports Traumatol Arthrosc. 2015;22(1):30–5. https://doi.org/10.1016/j.knee.2014.10.003. Epub 2014 Nov 20.
6. El-Kadiry AE, Lumbao C, Salame N, et al. Bone marrow aspirate concentrate versus platelet-rich plasma for treating knee osteoarthritis. BMC Musculoskelet Disord. 2022;23:23.

## Suggested Readings

Andia I, Maffulli N. Mesenchymal stromal cell products for intra-articular knee injections: from composition to product regulation. Ther Adv Musculoskelet Dis. 2021;13:1759720X20963618.

Barry F, Murphy M. Mesenchymal stem cells in joint disease and repair. Nat Rev Rheumatol. 2013;9(10):584–94.

Bruno S, et al. Mesenchymal stem cell-derived microvesicles protect against acute tubular injury. J Am Soc Nephrol. 2009;20(5):1053–67.

Caplan AI, Correa D. The MSC: an injury drugstore. Cell Stem Cell. 2011;9(1):11–5.

Chahla J, et al. Bone marrow aspirate concentrate for the treatment of osteoarthritis and other musculoskeletal conditions: a systematic review. Arthroscopy. 2016;32(5):969–81.

Filardo G, et al. Mesenchymal stem cells for the treatment of cartilage lesions: from preclinical findings to clinical application in orthopaedics. Knee Surg Sports Traumatol Arthrosc. 2010;18(4):504–17.

Gupta A, Cai X, Singh A, Kumar P, Liu J, Zhang X. Exosomes derived from mesenchymal stem cells: a new therapeutic approach to musculoskeletal diseases. Cell Tissue Res. 2017;368(3):421–433.

Granero-Moltó F, et al. Regenerative effects of transplanted mesenchymal stem cells in fracture healing. Stem Cells. 2009;27(8):1887–98.

Karp JM, Leng Teo GS. Mesenchymal stem cell homing: the devil is in the details. Cell Stem Cell. 2009;4(3):206–16.

Kim YS, et al. Clinical application of mesenchymal stem cells in the treatment of tendon and ligament injuries. Curr Stem Cell Res Ther. 2015;10(6):506–12.

Lai RC, et al. Exosome secreted by MSC reduces myocardial ischemia/reperfusion injury. Stem Cell Res. 2010;4(3):214–22.

López-Otín C, Blasco MA, Partridge L, Serrano M, Kroemer G. The hallmarks of aging. Cell. 2013a;153(6):1194–217.

López-Otín C, et al. The hallmarks of aging. Cell. 2013b;153(6):1194–217.

Phinney DG, Pittenger MF. Concise review: MSC-derived exosomes for cell-free therapy. Stem Cells. 2017;35(4):851–8.

Pittenger MF, et al. Multilineage potential of adult human mesenchymal stem cells. Science. 1999;284(5411):143–7.

Stolzing A, Jones E, McGonagle D, Scutt A. Age-related changes in human bone marrow-derived mesenchymal stem cells: consequences for cell therapies. Rejuvenation Res. 2008a;11(5):719–32.

Stolzing A, et al. Age-related changes in human bone marrow-derived mesenchymal stem cells: consequences for cell therapies. Rejuvenation Res. 2008b;11(5):837–45.

Strand N, et al. STEP guidelines for regenerative medicine: knee osteoarthritis. American Society of Pain and Neuroscience (ASPN); 2022;15:2683–2745. https://doi.org/10.2147/JPR.S370469.

Uysal AC, Mizuno H. Tendon regeneration and repair with adipose derived stem cells. Curr Stem Cell Res Ther. 2010;5(2):161–7.

Yin K, Wang S, Zhao RC. Exosomes from mesenchymal stem/stromal cells: a new therapeutic paradigm. Biomark Res. 2019;7:8.

# Exosomes and Extravesicles

# 6

Ripu D. Arora

Exosomes are nanoscale extracellular vesicles that have emerged as potential key players in the field of regenerative medicine, particularly for their role in managing pain and promoting tissue healing. These microscopic, membrane-bound particles are released by various cell types, notably MSCs, and act as intercellular messengers, delivering bioactive molecules to target cells.

At present, exosome-based therapies remain investigational and are not yet approved by the FDA in the United States. However, as delivery platforms improve and research expands, they are poised to become an important addition to regenerative and interventional pain medicine.

## 6.1 Structure and Composition of Exosomes

Exosomes are nano-sized extracellular vesicles ranging from 30 to 150 nm in diameter. These vesicles are formed through the endosomal pathway and are released when multivesicular bodies (MVBs) fuse with the plasma membrane.

### 6.1.1 Composition

The exosomal membrane is composed of a lipid bilayer, enriched with cholesterol, sphingomyelin, ceramide, and lipid raft-associated proteins. These components confer structural stability and facilitate exosome formation and trafficking.

Exosomes are rich in a variety of therapeutic cargo. This includes cytokines, growth factors, enzymes, mRNA and microRNA, lipids, and proteins.

R. D. Arora (✉)
Arora Pain Clinic, Torrance, CA, USA



R. D. Arora (ed.), *Regenerative Medicine in Pain Practice*,
https://doi.org/10.1007/978-3-032-22644-0_6

This molecular payload enables exosomes to influence the local cellular environment at the site of tissue injury or inflammation, facilitating repair and regeneration. The events involve Inflammation resolution, angiogenesis, neuronal repair, and pain signal modulation.

### 6.1.2 Unique Surface Markers

Exosomes can be distinguished from other extracellular vesicles (EVs) by their surface proteins, especially a conserved set of Cluster of Differentiation (CD) markers:

CD9, CD63, CD81: Members of the tetraspanin family; these are commonly used for identification and isolation of exosomes.
TSG101, Alix: Involved in ESCRT (Endosomal Sorting Complex Required for Transport) machinery, indicating an endosomal origin.

These markers play an essential role in experimental identification and are frequently employed in techniques such as immuno-isolation, flow cytometry, and Western blot analysis. They play roles in membrane organization and protein sorting.

### 6.1.3 Cargo Diversity and Cell-Type Specificity

The most intriguing aspect of exosomes is their cargo, which reflects the physiological or pathological state of the parent cell. This cargo is packaged selectively and it includes the following (Fig. 6.1):

**Nucleic Acids**
MicroRNA (miRNA)
Messenger RNA (mRNA)
Transfer RNA (tRNA)
Mitochondrial DNA (mtDNA)
Circular RNA (circRNA)
Long non-coding RNA (lncRNA)
Double-stranded DNA (dsDNA) and single-stranded DNA (ssDNA)

**Proteins**
Heat shock proteins (HSP70, HSP90), Alix, TSG101
Cytoskeletal elements
Signaling molecules
Cytokines with anti-apoptotic, mitogenic, anti-scarring, or angiogenic functions

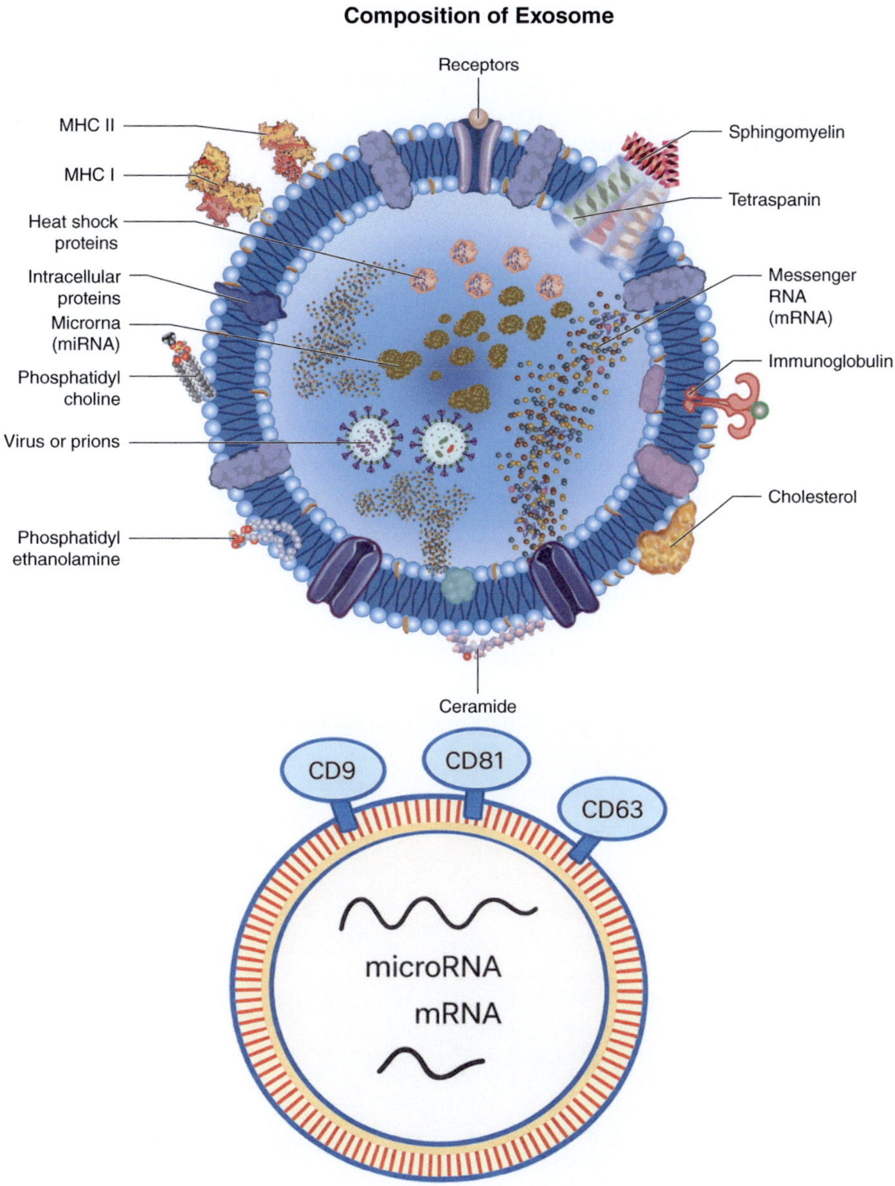


**Fig. 6.1** Extracellular vesicles are membrane-bound particles composed of a lipid bilayer and a diverse molecular cargo. Surface proteins commonly include tetraspanins such as CD9, CD63, and CD81, which are frequently used as extracellular vesicle markers. Intravascular contents include nucleic acids, such as microRNA and messenger RNA (mRNA), as well as proteins and bioactive lipids. These components contribute to intercellular communication and modulation of recipient cell behavior

**Lipids**

Ceramide (involved in membrane curvature and cargo sorting).

Sphingomyelin, cholesterol, and phosphatidylserine which contribute to membrane stability and fusion competency.

This cargo is not randomly distributed. It is cell-type specific and dynamically changes in response to the cell's microenvironment, such as inflammation, hypoxia, or injury. Thus, exosomes serve as miniature messengers delivering instructions from one cell to another. This cargo is functionally active and can be transferred to recipient cells for modulation of gene expression and cellular behavior.

## 6.2 Mechanisms of Action

Once released, exosomes travel to the site of injury, where they interact with damaged cells and modulate cellular activity. Their therapeutic effects include the following (Fig. 6.2):

Reduction in pain and inflammation
Promotion of cell proliferation
Suppression of apoptosis (cell death)
Inhibition of fibrosis
Enhancement of angiogenesis (formation of new blood vessels)

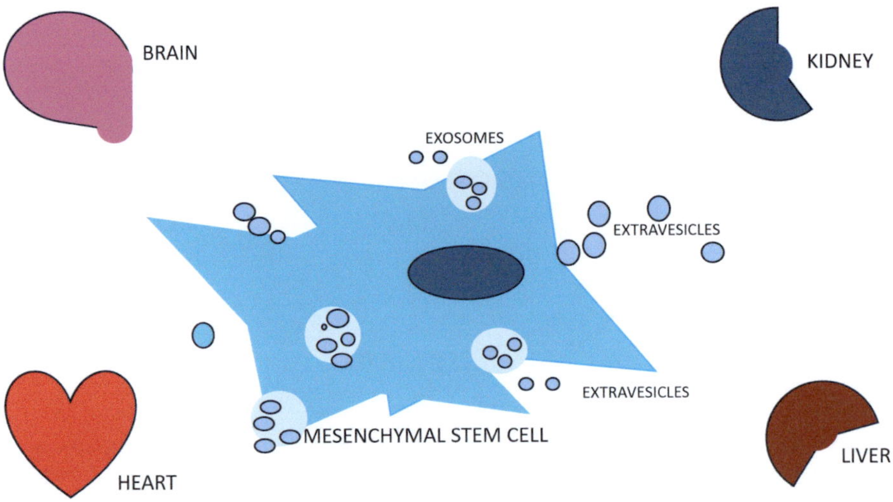


**Fig. 6.2** Exosomes released from mesenchymal stem cells (MSCs) interact with various organs (brain, heart, liver, kidney), mediating repair by reducing apoptosis, suppressing inflammation, and promoting cell proliferation and regeneration. The image highlights the broad regenerative capabilities of exosomes across different tissues

These mechanisms make exosomes a powerful tool in treating a range of conditions, including musculoskeletal injuries, neurodegenerative diseases, and organ damage.

## 6.3 Exosome Effect on Various Organs

*Brain*: Exosomes confer long-term neuroprotection, increase cell proliferation, suppress inflammation, and promote functional recovery.

*Heart*: They contribute to reduced infarction size, suppression of inflammation, enhanced formation of blood vessels, and overall improved cardiac function.

*Kidney*: Exosome therapy results in reduced fibrosis, inhibition of necrosis, and enhanced cell proliferation.

*Liver*: The benefits include reduced oxidative stress, suppression of inflammation, improved functional recovery, and decreased liver injury.

## 6.4 Biogenesis of Exosomes

Exosomes are a subtype of extracellular vesicles that originate from the endosomal system within cells. Their biogenesis is a tightly regulated, multi-step process that begins with the formation of early endosomes and culminates in the release of mature exosomes into the extracellular environment.

### 6.4.1 Initiation of Exosome Biogenesis

The process begins when a signaling cell releases molecular signals such as exosomes, small bioactive molecules, or other extracellular vesicles that interact with specific receptors located on the plasma membrane of a responding cell. These receptors are embedded within the outer layer of the cell membrane and serve as molecular sensors to detect environmental cues or intercellular messages.

### 6.4.2 Formation of Early Endosomes

The invaginated portion of the plasma membrane progressively deepens and eventually pinches off to form a distinct intracellular structure known as an early endosome**.** This is a membrane-bound vesicle with a bilayer lipid membrane, indicating its origin from the cell's plasma membrane (Fig. 6.3).

Notably, during this invagination process, the outer layer of the parent cell's plasma membrane becomes the inner layer of the newly formed early endosome. This topological inversion is critical because it preserves the orientation of surface proteins and receptors in a manner that enables the sorting and eventual secretion of functional exosomes.

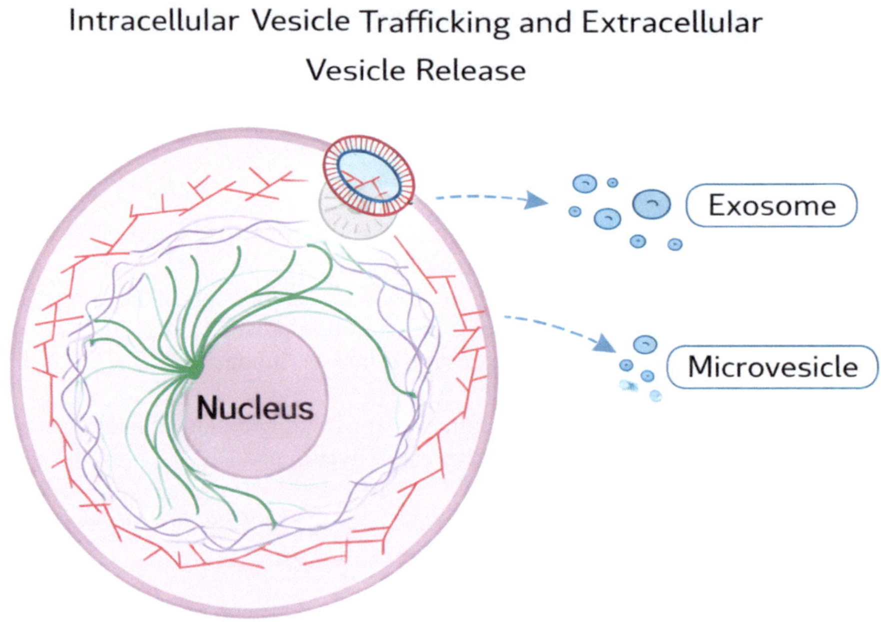


**Fig. 6.3** Early endosome intracellular structure and vesicle release in a mesenchymal stem cell

Schematic representation of a mesenchymal stem cell showing the nucleus, cytoskeletal framework, and plasma membrane. The highlighted membrane region illustrates vesicle budding and release, which generates extracellular vesicles that mediate paracrine signaling, immune modulation, angiogenesis, and tissue regeneration.

### 6.4.3 Interaction with Cellular Organelles

As early endosomes mature, they interact with other cellular organelles, including the Golgi apparatus, mitochondria, and the endoplasmic reticulum (ER) to exchange molecular cargo. These interactions are critical for the functional enrichment of the endosomes, as they incorporate various proteins, lipids, and nucleic acids that will eventually be packaged into exosomes.

### 6.4.4 Formation of Intraluminal Vesicles (ILVs)

The early endosomes gradually transition into *late endosomes*, a maturation step characterized by the formation of intraluminal vesicles (ILVs). ILVs are created through inward budding and invagination of the limiting membrane of the early endosome. This process results in the sequestration of cytosolic components (the jelly-like fluid component of the cytoplasm containing water, ions, and soluble proteins crucial for metabolism) within small vesicles inside the larger endosomal body (Fig. 6.4).

Notably, the inner membrane of each ILV is derived from the outer endosomal membrane, which itself contains elements of the parent cell's plasma membrane. As a result, ILVs often carry specific membrane proteins and lipids reflective of their cellular origin.

### 6.4.5 Multivesicular Bodies (MVBs) Maturation and Potential Exosome Release

Late endosomes containing numerous ILVs are referred to as multivesicular bodies (MVBs). These MVBs represent a critical decision point in the exosome pathway. They can either fuse with lysosomes for degradation of their contents or merge with the plasma membrane of the cell, leading to the release of ILVs into the extracellular space as exosomes.

This entire process is a highly regulated point in exosome biology and is crucial for cellular homeostasis and communication, as exosomes play key roles in intercellular signaling, immune response modulation, and the spread of pathogenic proteins in various diseases.

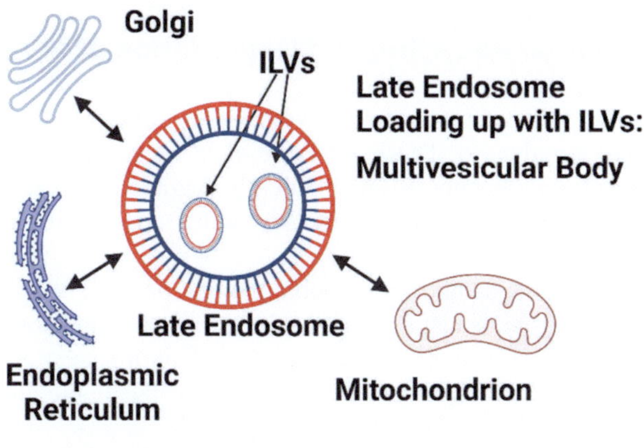


**Fig. 6.4** Biogenesis and release of exosomes from mesenchymal stem cells. Schematic representation of intracellular vesicle formation showing contributions from the Golgi apparatus, endoplasmic reticulum, and mitochondria for the generation of multivesicular bodies. Fusion of these compartments with the plasma membrane releases exosomes that mediate intercellular communication, immune modulation, angiogenesis, and tissue regeneration

### 6.4.6 Directed Transport and Docking of MVBs

MVBs are transported through the cytoplasm along microtubules via the cytoskeletal network, using motor proteins such as kinesin and dynein. This trafficking is not random but directed toward specific plasma membrane docking sites, where MVBs interact with tethering and fusion machinery, including SNARE proteins and Rab GTPases. These interactions ensure that the MVBs are properly aligned and prepared for membrane fusion.

### 6.4.7 Fusion with the Plasma Membrane and Exosome Release

Upon reaching the plasma membrane, MVBs undergo membrane fusion, a process mediated by protein complexes that allow the outer membrane of the MVB to integrate with the cell's inner plasma membrane. This fusion event leads to the release of the intraluminal vesicles (ILVs) into the extracellular space. Once outside the cell, these ILVs are referred to as exosomes.

*Exosomes are typically 30–150 nm* in diameter and carry a cargo reflective of their endosomal original proteins, lipids, RNA, and DNA. These vesicles serve as intercellular communicators, delivering their contents to recipient cells either locally or at a distance via bodily fluids.

## 6.5 Intracellular Recycling and Degradation of MVBs

Not all MVBs are destined for exosome secretion. A subset of MVBs is rerouted toward degradation pathways. These MVBs marked for recycling are delivered to lysosomes, where their contents are enzymatically degraded. This pathway is essential for intracellular quality control, especially under stress conditions or nutrient deprivation.

Additionally, autophagosomes, the double-membrane vesicles that engulf damaged organelles and proteins can fuse with MVBs to form amphisomes, which also ultimately merge with lysosomes for degradation. This intersection of autophagy and the endosomal system highlight the dynamic and adaptable nature of vesicle trafficking (Fig. 6.5).

This tightly controlled balance ensures that cells can modulate communication, signaling, and waste disposal as needed, with significant implications for development, immunity, and disease.

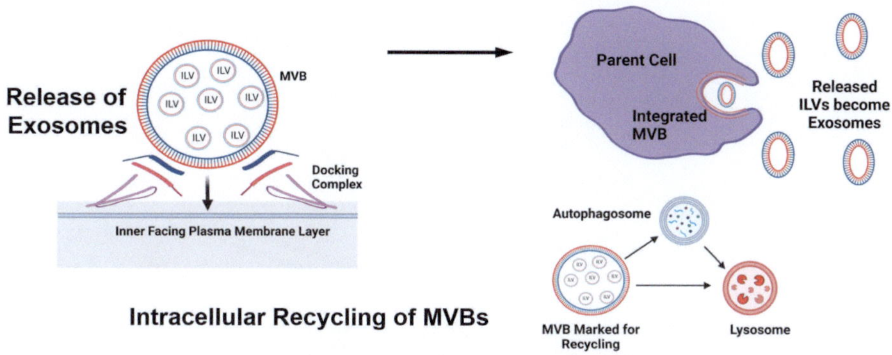


**Fig. 6.5** Biogenesis of exosomes. Exosomes originate as intraluminal vesicles within multivesicular bodies (MVBs). When MVBs fuse with the plasma membrane, these vesicles are released as exosomes into the extracellular space to mediate intercellular communication. Alternatively, MVBs can be directed to lysosomes for degradation and intracellular recycling

## 6.6 Therapeutic Applications of Extracellular Vesicles in Regenerative Pain Medicine

EVs, including exosomes and microvesicles, have emerged as key mediators of intercellular communication with significant implications for regenerative medicine and clinical pain practice. These nano-sized, membrane-bound particles are secreted by various cell types and carry a cargo of proteins, lipids, and nucleic acids, enabling them to influence target cells locally and systemically.

In the context of pain and tissue degeneration, EVs offer a novel therapeutic platform capable of modifying the cellular microenvironment, modulating immune responses, and promoting tissue regeneration. Their pleiotropic functions align with several key cellular targets and mechanisms relevant to chronic pain syndromes, degenerative joint disease, and neuropathic injury.

### 6.6.1 Functions of EVs (Fig. 6.6)

**Diagnostics**

EVs and exosomes contain molecular signatures that mirror the state of their parent cells. This includes proteins, lipids, and nucleic acids (e.g., microRNAs, DNA fragments), making them valuable as noninvasive biomarkers for the following:

- Cancer detection
- Neurodegenerative diseases
- Inflammatory conditions
- Metabolic syndromes

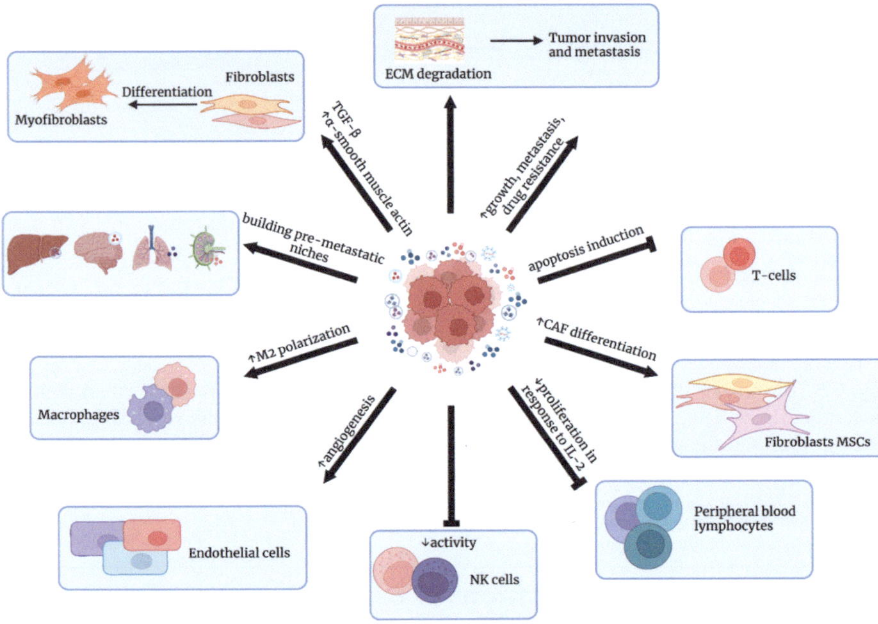


**Fig. 6.6** Functions of exosomes

**Therapeutics**

As natural carriers of bioactive molecules, EVs serve as vehicles for targeted drug delivery, enhancing therapeutic precision while minimizing systemic side effects.

Due to their natural role in molecular transport and their ability to cross biological barriers (e.g., blood-brain barriers), exosomes serve as nanocarriers.

**Exosomes as Nanocarriers**

- Drug delivery (e.g., chemotherapeutics, RNA therapeutics)
- Gene editing tools (e.g., CRISPR/Cas9 components)
- Anti-inflammatory and anti-scarring agents
- Regenerative Medicine: EVs promote tissue repair by transferring regenerative signals, such as growth factors and miRNAs, to local or distant cells involved in the healing processes.
- Exosomes derived from MSCs and other regenerative cell types promote angiogenesis, neurogenesis, fibroblast migration, wound healing, and modulation of chronic inflammation.

## 6.6.2 Mechanisms and Clinical Correlates

EVs interact with a wide range of cell types, supporting regenerative outcomes through the following mechanisms:

**Fibroblast-to-Myofibroblast Differentiation:**
EVs promote fibroblast activation and matrix remodeling, critical for restoring tissue structure in degenerative conditions such as tendinopathy or post-surgical healing.

**Tissue Priming and Niche Conditioning:**
EVs may "precondition" tissues analogous to preparing pre-metastatic niches in oncology—by enhancing local receptivity to regenerative inputs, useful in managing ischemic or fibrotic tissues.

**Macrophage Polarization:**
EVs facilitate the shift of macrophages toward an M2 phenotype, reducing chronic inflammation and supporting tissue regeneration, key functions in osteoarthritis and intervertebral disc disease.

**Angiogenesis:**
By acting on endothelial cells, EVs promote neovascularization, essential for oxygenation and nutrient delivery in compromised tissues such as diabetic ulcers or avascular necrosis.

**Immune Modulation:**
EVs can dampen overactive immune responses by reducing natural killer (NK) cell activity and promoting T cell apoptosis or tolerance, thereby attenuating autoimmunity and neuroinflammation.

**Stem Cell and Stromal Cell Activation:**
EVs support MSC proliferation and differentiation, crucial for joint and connective tissue regeneration.

**Matrix Remodeling:**
By influencing extracellular matrix (ECM) turnover, EVs contribute to tissue repair while potentially preventing pathological fibrosis.

**Therapeutic Cargo Delivery:**
EVs can be engineered or enriched with anti-inflammatory agents, mRNAs, or miRNAs to further enhance their reparative capacity.

### 6.6.3 Clinical Applications in Pain Medicine

*Intercellular Communication*: EVs mediate transfer of therapeutic signals across cell types, aiding in coordinated tissue repair.

*Immune Modulation*: They mitigate neuroinflammatory processes underlying conditions such as CRPS or radiculopathy.

*Waste Management*: EVs assist in the clearance of cellular debris and metabolic byproducts, improving tissue homeostasis.

## 6.7 Conclusion

Incorporating EVs into pain practice represents a frontier in regenerative therapeutics, offering cell-free alternatives with low immunogenicity and high clinical utility. As research advances, their integration into protocols for musculoskeletal pain, neuropathy, and postoperative recovery holds promise for transforming outcomes into precision pain medicine.

## 6.8 Clinical Applications of Exosomes in Musculoskeletal and Neural Pain Syndromes

Their application in musculoskeletal and neural pain syndromes is supported by preclinical evidence and early clinical observations, highlighting their potential as a cell-free, biologically active therapeutic strategy. Below are condition-specific mechanisms by which exosomes contribute to pain relief and functional recovery.

### 6.8.1 Osteoarthritis (OA)

**Cartilage Regeneration**
Exosomes derived from MSCs deliver an array of anabolic factors, including chondroprotective microRNAs and anti-apoptotic proteins, to native chondrocytes. These vesicles stimulate chondrocyte proliferation, enhance ECM synthesis, and inhibit catabolic, cartilage degrading enzymes such as matrix metalloproteinases. The result is restoration of cartilage homeostasis and attenuation of structural degradation.

**Synovial Inflammation Modulation**
Exosomes downregulate pro-inflammatory cytokines like IL-1β and TNF-α and modulate synoviocyte behavior to suppress chronic synovitis. By altering the inflammatory milieu of the joint, they help preserve joint integrity and delay OA progression.

**Perfect Union**
Through the mechanisms listed above, exosomes decrease joint effusions by shifting the environment from one of destructive inflammation and synoviocyte irritation to one of regenerative healing, less pain and improved mobility.

### 6.8.2 Tendon Injuries

**Tendon Healing Enhancement**

Exosomes influence tendon biology by promoting tenocyte proliferation, differentiation, and collagen organization. They also facilitate ECM remodeling and contribute to restoration of tendon architecture and tensile strength. These mechanisms support both acute and chronic tendon repair, offering a biologic adjunct to traditional physical therapy or surgical interventions.

Exosomes have been shown to activate tenogenic differentiation pathways, enhance tenocyte proliferation and migration, and regulate macrophage phenotypes toward a regenerative M2 profile. These actions collectively reduce proinflammatory cytokine production, fibrosis, and cell apoptosis, creating a conducive environment for tendon repair.

Growth Factors & Pathways: TGF-β, PTEN, AMOT/Fgf-B1, SMAD3/5, PI3K/AKT, MAPK/ERK1/2
miRNAs: miR-21, miR-29, miR-221, miR-210

PEP + TISSEEL matrices and IFNγ-primed MSC-derived exosomes have demonstrated enhanced tendon regeneration.

Engineered exosomes from human umbilical MSCs (HUMSCs) carrying miR-21a-3p have shown accelerated tendon healing in vivo.

### 6.8.3 Skeletal Muscle Injuries

**Myogenic Stimulation and Fibrosis Reduction**

In muscle injury models, exosomes have been shown to activate satellite cells, increase myofiber formation, promote angiogenesis, and polarize macrophages to the M2 phenotype suppressing fibrotic pathways. This leads to accelerated regeneration. Additionally, they mitigate muscle fibrosis and reduce apoptosis of myoblasts, leading to improved structural and functional outcomes.

Their potential use spans from acute sports injuries to chronic conditions like sarcopenia or muscular dystrophies.

This is achieved through its cargo using miRNAs: miR-494, miR-126, miR-230, miR-486-5p, and signaling molecules: FoxO1, Neuregulin-1 (NRG-1).

### 6.8.4 Bone Repair

**Promotion of Osteogenesis**

Exosomes interact with osteoblasts and osteoclasts, supporting bone matrix production and mineralization while maintaining physiological bone turnover. They provide a paracrine stimulus that enhances fracture healing, improves graft incorporation, and reduces the need for synthetic implants or bone morphogenetic proteins.

### 6.8.5 Peripheral Nerve Injuries

**Neuroregeneration and Functional Recovery**

MSC-derived exosomes enhance neurogenesis by promoting the expression of myelin-associated and neurogenic genes, increasing Schwann cell proliferation and migration, stimulating neurite outgrowth, and improving local vascularization. A balanced M1/M2 macrophage response is also achieved, contributing to reduced neuroinflammation and enhanced axonal repair.

Nucleic acid components in neurogenesis include miRNAs: miR-21, miR-222, miR-26b, miR-132, miR-210, along with proteins like Kon2/PI3K/AKT, Wnt/β--catenin, SOX2, PTEN.

Exosome use is being explored in neuropathic pain syndromes, nerve compression injuries, and post-surgical neurorepair. These effects are critical in reducing chronic pain and restoring sensory and motor function.

PEP-exosome combination systems and ExoNT-3D nerve guidance conduits (NGCs) replicate the architecture of native nerve tissue, supporting directed axonal regeneration.

## 6.9 Advantages of Exosome Therapy in Soft Tissue Regeneration

- Cell-Free Therapy: Low immunogenicity and low risk of tumor formation, unlike live cell transplants.
- Scalability and Stability: Exosomes can be mass-produced, stored long-term, and standardized for clinical use.
- Customizability: The miRNA and protein cargo of exosomes can be engineered to target specific molecular pathways or disease states.
- Injectable Format: Easily administered in outpatient settings using image-guided procedures for localized treatment.
- Clinical and Preclinical Insights.
- Engineered exosomes such as miR-21a-3p-enriched HUMSC-Exos have demonstrated accelerated healing in tendon injury models.
- IFNγ-primed MSC exosomes exhibit enhanced immunomodulatory effects, optimizing the regenerative microenvironment.
- Milk-derived EVs, a novel noninvasive source, have shown regenerative efficacy in muscle and tendon models, expanding the potential pool of therapeutic EVs.

## 6.10 Exosome Sources in Research

The following sources have demonstrated robust regenerative capacity in various preclinical models of muscle injury:

Urine-derived stem cell EVs (USC-EVs), Bovine milk-derived EVs, Gingiva-derived and adipose-derived stem cell exosomes (G-ADSC-Exos).

## 6.11 Clinical Outlook and Future Directions

The incorporation of exosome-based therapies into regenerative pain practice offers multiple clinical advantages:

- Opioid-Sparing Effect: Through biologic modulation of inflammation and tissue repair, exosomes may reduce reliance on analgesics, particularly opioids.
- Minimally Invasive: As injectable, cell-free products, exosomes offer a nonsurgical option for a range of degenerative and traumatic conditions.
- Personalized Therapy: The potential for patient-specific or disease-targeted exosome preparations opens the door to precision regenerative medicine.
- Multi-tissue Applications: Their ability to act across joint, muscle, tendon, bone, and nerve tissues makes exosomes uniquely versatile in clinical pain management.

## 6.12 Conclusion

Exosome research continues to advance rapidly, and their potential role in musculoskeletal and neural pain syndromes is becoming increasingly significant. Unlike traditional cellular therapies, exosomes offer the ability to modulate cell behavior, regulate immune responses, and support tissue repair with fewer complications.

Evidence from preclinical and early clinical studies suggests that MSC-derived exosomes improve pain, function, and structural recovery, particularly in conditions such as osteoarthritis. Their anti-inflammatory and regenerative properties, combined with low immunogenicity and toxicity, make them promising for patients with common comorbidities like obesity, diabetes, hypertension, and cardiovascular disease.

Importantly, safety profiles are consistently favorable, with few reported adverse effects and no significant drug interactions. Clinical trials, including dose-escalation studies using umbilical cord MSC-derived exosomes, show good tolerance and biocompatibility across diverse patient populations.

Despite these encouraging findings, long-term safety data and larger clinical trials are still needed. Standardized protocols, mechanistic studies, and careful monitoring of inflammatory and metabolic markers will be critical for ensuring consistent and effective outcomes.

## Suggested Readings

Abdulmalek OAAY, Husain KH, AlKhalifa HKAA, et al. MSC-derived exosomes in orthopedic disorders: emerging clinical evidence. Int J Mol Sci. 2024;25(6):3562.

Alcaraz MJ, Compañ A, Guillén MI. Extracellular vesicles from mesenchymal stem cells as novel treatments for musculoskeletal diseases. Cells. 2019;9(1):98.

Andreu Z, Yáñez-Mó M. Tetraspanins in extracellular vesicle formation and function. Front Immunol. 2014;5:442. https://doi.org/10.3389/fimmu.2014.00442.

Chen L, Xiang B, Wang X, Zheng G. Exosomes derived from tendon stem cells promote tendon healing by modulating inflammation and collagen synthesis. Stem Cell Res Ther. 2018;9(1):7.

Cosenza S, Ruiz M, Toupet K, et al. Mesenchymal stem cell-derived exosomes protect cartilage and bone from degradation in osteoarthritis. Sci Rep. 2017;7:16214.

Gerami MH, Khorram R, Rasoolzadegan S, et al. Clinical safety and efficacy of exosome therapies in musculoskeletal disorders: a systematic review. Eur J Med Res. 2023;28(1):86.

José Alcaraz M. Exosome-based therapies in degenerative joint disease. Biochem Pharmacol. 2024;228:116226.

Kalluri R, LeBleu VS. The biology, function, and biomedical applications of exosomes. Science. 2020;367(6478):eaau6977. https://doi.org/10.1126/science.aau6977.

Ling MTM, Govindaraju K, Lokanathan Y, et al. Exosome-based therapeutics in musculoskeletal regeneration. Cell Biochem Funct. 2023;41(8):1044–59.

Mendt M, Rezvani K, Shpall E. MSC-derived exosomes as a cell-free therapy for musculoskeletal diseases. Trends Mol Med. 2019;25(10):869–82.

Ren S, Wang C, Guo S. Advances in mesenchymal stem cell-derived exosomes for osteoarthritis therapy. Med Sci Monit. 2022;28:e935937.

Ryan ST, Hosseini-Beheshti E, Afrose D, et al. MSC exosomes in regenerative orthopedics: mechanisms and translational potential. Int J Mol Sci. 2021;22(6):3023.

Sankaranarayanan J, Kim HK, Kang JY, et al. Mesenchymal stem cell-derived exosomes in cartilage repair: new insights. Int J Mol Sci. 2025;26(12):5447.

Vadhan A, Gupta T, Hsu WL. Therapeutic applications of exosomes in regenerative medicine. Int J Mol Sci. 2024;25(17):9149.

Valadi H, Ekström K, Bossios A, Sjöstrand M, Lee JJ, Lötvall JO. Exosome-mediated transfer of mRNAs and microRNAs is a novel mechanism of genetic exchange between cells. Nat Cell Biol. 2007;9(6):654–9. https://doi.org/10.1038/ncb1596.

van Niel G, D'Angelo G, Raposo G. Shedding light on the cell biology of extracellular vesicles. Nat Rev Mol Cell Biol. 2018;19(4):213–28.

Wang Y, Kong Y, Du J, et al. Clinical potential of exosomes in musculoskeletal disorders: a translational perspective. J Transl Med. 2025;23(1):641.

Yáñez-Mó M, Siljander PRM, Andreu Z, Zavec AB, Borràs FE, Buzas EI, et al. Biological properties of extracellular vesicles and their physiological functions. J Extracell Vesicles. 2015;4(1):27066.

# Regenerative Cell Protein Arrays in Pain Management and Musculoskeletal Diseases

7

Joseph Cabaret and Ripu D. Arora

## 7.1 Introduction

Regenerative cell protein arrays (RCPAs) represent an innovative, cell-free therapeutic platform derived from placental mesenchymal stem cells (MSCs). Designed to leverage the regenerative potential of the MSC secretome, RCPAs deliver a reproducible and quantifiable blend of signaling molecules cytokines, growth factors, and RNAs that promote soft tissue and joint repair. This next-generation approach offers clinicians a scalable, low-risk, and biologically potent alternative to conventional cell-based or platelet-derived therapies.

## 7.2 Mechanism of Action: Paracrine Signaling over Cellular Differentiation

Contemporary research confirms that MSCs exert their therapeutic effects primarily via paracrine mechanisms rather than direct tissue integration or differentiation. The MSC secretome including soluble factors and extracellular vesicles (EVs) modulates local inflammation, recruits progenitor cells, stimulates angiogenesis, and facilitates matrix remodeling across musculoskeletal tissues (Fig. 7.1).

In preclinical models, MSC-derived EVs and conditioned media have accelerated healing in muscle and tendon injuries. Notably, microRNA (miRNA) cargoes such as miR-494 are implicated in reducing fibrosis, enhancing biomechanical strength, and shortening recovery timelines.

J. Cabaret
Pain Clinic Camarillo, Camarillo, CA, USA

R. D. Arora (✉)
Arora Pain Clinic, Torrance, CA, USA



R. D. Arora (ed.), *Regenerative Medicine in Pain Practice*,
https://doi.org/10.1007/978-3-032-22644-0_7

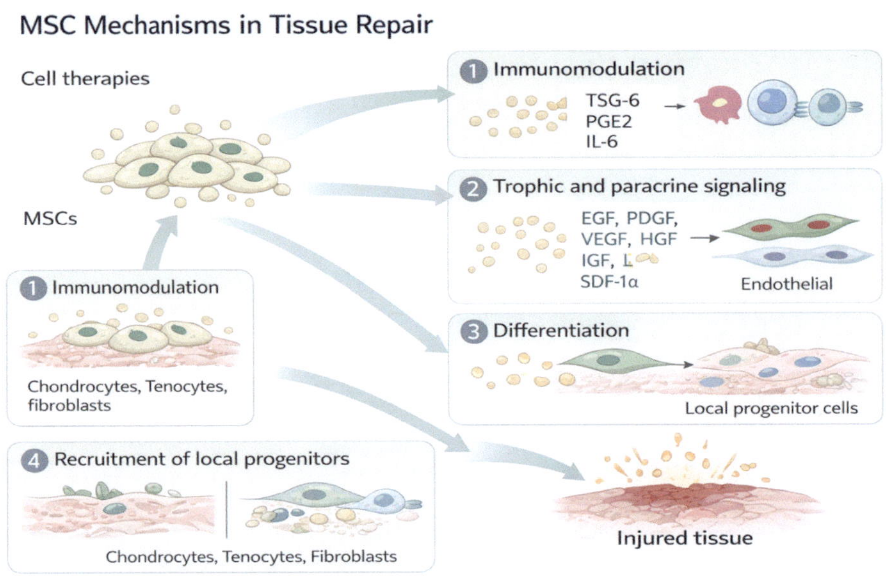


**Fig. 7.1** Regenerative functions of cells

## 7.3 Bioreactor Production and Molecular Quantification

RCPAs are manufactured in controlled bioreactor environments using placental tissue sourced from multiple compartments (e.g., amnion, chorion, umbilical cord). This method standardizes the secretion of therapeutic molecules including miRNA, messenger RNA (mRNA), long non-coding RNA (lncRNA), cytokines, and growth factors, producing a cell-free, DNA-free therapeutic solution.

The bioreactor process allows for precise quantification of bioactive ingredients, minimizing the variability seen in traditional secretome products that depend on donor variability or culture conditions. As a result, clinicians gain access to a highly reproducible and customizable regenerative tool.

## 7.4 Comparative Potency and Safety Profile

Compared to autologous biologics such as platelet-rich plasma (PRP), RCPAs offer a more comprehensive regenerative signaling platform. While PRP is often limited to a narrow profile of growth factors, RCPAs mimic the full spectrum of the MSC secretome. Preclinical data indicate that secretome-based products may even surpass cell-based therapies in efficacy, with successful applications across osteoarthritis, tendon injury, and inflammatory conditions.

Importantly, because RCPAs are acellular and DNA-free, they avoid immunologic and oncogenic risks associated with transplanted or genetically unstable cells.

**Table 7.1** Regenerative protein array in MSK medicine

| Protein/cytokine | Function in MSK regeneration | Primary biological source |
|---|---|---|
| Platelet-derived growth factor (PDGF) | Stimulates cellular proliferation and angiogenesis | PRP, platelet lysates |
| Transforming growth factor-β (TGF-β) | Regulates inflammation, promotes extracellular matrix (ECM) synthesis | PRP, bone marrow aspirate concentrate (BMAC) |
| Vascular endothelial growth factor (VEGF) | Induces neovascularization and tissue perfusion | PRP, BMAC |
| Insulin-like growth factor-1 (IGF-1) | Enhances cartilage and bone matrix formation | Plasma, BMAC |
| Fibroblast growth factor-2 (FGF-2) | Supports tendon, ligament, and connective tissue healing | PRP, BMAC |
| Interleukin-1 receptor antagonist protein (IRAP) | Blocks IL-1β activity, reducing joint and soft tissue inflammation | Autologous conditioned serum |
| Alpha-2 macroglobulin (A2M) | Inhibits cartilage-degrading enzymes (e.g., MMPs) | Plasma, PRP |
| Hepatocyte growth factor (HGF) | Exerts anti-inflammatory effects and promotes cellular regeneration | BMAC, adipose tissue |
| Matrix metalloproteinase inhibitors | Prevent degradation of cartilage ECM | Plasma-derived proteins |
| TNF-α blockers | Modulate chronic inflammatory cascades | IRAP, plasma fractions |
| $PGE_2$ | Immune modulation, analgesic effect | Bone marrow and adipose MSCs |
| TSG-6 | ECM stabilization, anti-inflammatory | MSCs from all compartments |
| Galectin-1, Galectin-3 | Anti-fibrotic, immune modulation | MSCs and placental tissues |
| Stromal-derived factor-1 (SDF-1) | Stem cell recruitment | Bone marrow MSCs |

Multiple studies support their low immunogenicity, absence of tumorigenicity, and superior safety profile. The RCPA has the Protein/cytokine profile as in listed table below (Table 7.1).

## 7.5 Customization and Clinical Delivery Strategies

RCPA formulations can be tailored to specific clinical targets, such as:

- Anti-inflammatory arrays for inflammatory arthritis or autoimmune myopathies
- Pro-angiogenic profiles for avascular necrosis or chronic tendinopathy
- Matrix-remodeling support in rotator cuff pathology or ligament injury

*Delivery routes include the following*:

Local administration: Intra-articular injections, peritendinous delivery, or ultrasound-guided muscle/tendon injections

Systemic administration: Intravenous infusion in cases requiring broader immunomodulation
Combined protocols: For cases requiring both local and systemic regenerative effects

These strategies align with the natural distribution patterns of paracrine signaling, enhancing both specificity and efficacy.

## 7.6 Regulatory Classification and Safety Considerations

Due to their acellular and DNA-free nature, RCPAs do not fall under the FDA's HCT/P (Human Cell and Tissue Product) regulations, allowing a regulatory pathway akin to nutraceuticals or biologics. This classification reduces regulatory burdens while maintaining product safety and consistency.

Their non-cellular formulation eliminates concerns of immune rejection, tumor formation, or genetic instability, making RCPAs a highly safe and scalable therapeutic option for clinical use.

## 7.7 Clinical Evidence and Future Research Directions

While human trials on placenta-derived secretome therapies are still emerging, the broader field of MSC-secretome research is expanding rapidly. Ongoing clinical studies are exploring the use of exosomes, EVs, and conditioned media in treating the following:

- Osteoarthritis
- Autoimmune disorders
- Post-surgical inflammation
- Chronic pain syndromes
- Pulmonary and cardiac fibrosis

Preclinical models continue to validate the regenerative impact of these products in soft tissue and orthopedic applications, such as rat models of tendon injury, cartilage repair, and muscle regeneration.

However, key challenges remain, including the following:

- Standardization of manufacturing protocols
- Long-term safety and efficacy evaluation
- Optimized dosing and frequency schedules

### 7.7.1 Discussion

This case illustrates the clinical utility of RCPA therapy in a nonoperative, degenerative tendon condition where traditional biologics (e.g., PRP) may offer limited durability. By delivering a broad spectrum of cytokines and regenerative signals, RCPA therapy facilitates resolution of chronic inflammation and supports soft tissue repair.

### 7.7.2 In Summary

RCPAs can be used in patients seeking a non-surgical, cell-free regenerative option.
Ideal for chronic tendinopathies where inflammation and failed healing predominate.
Requires ultrasound guidance and patient education to optimize outcomes.
Avoid concurrent anti-inflammatory medications that may blunt paracrine signaling.

The following is a structured list of musculoskeletal (MSK) diseases and conditions where RCPAs may offer clinical effectiveness, based on their mechanisms of action (e.g., anti-inflammatory, pro-angiogenic, ECM-modulating, immunomodulatory). Each condition includes a rationale for use and clinical relevance.

## 7.8 Clinical Application in Pain Management and MSK Diseases

### 7.8.1 Osteoarthritis (OA)

**Target** Articular cartilage, synovial membrane

**Mechanism**

Suppression of inflammatory cytokines (e.g., IL-1β, TNF-α)
Promotion of chondrogenesis via TGF-β, IGF-1
Preservation of cartilage matrix integrity (e.g., TIMP, TSG-6)

**Clinical Relevance**

Delays progression of OA
Reduces pain and stiffness
Enhances joint function as a non-surgical alternative

### 7.8.2 Tendinopathies (e.g., Rotator Cuff, Achilles, Patellar)

**Target** Degenerative tendons

**Mechanism**
Stimulates tenocyte proliferation and collagen remodeling
Reduces matrix-degrading enzymes (MMPs)
Modulates local immune responses (↑ M2 macrophages, ↓ M1 cytokines)

**Clinical Relevance**
Facilitates tendon healing without surgery
Improves tendon load-bearing and tensile strength
Complements physical therapy and eccentric loading

### 7.8.3 Muscle Injuries and Myopathies

**Target** Skeletal muscle fibers and satellite cells

**Mechanism**
Enhances myogenesis (via miR-494, IGF-1, NRG-1)
Reduces fibrosis and inflammation
Promotes angiogenesis and muscle regeneration

**Clinical Relevance**
Accelerates healing in sports injuries
Useful in sarcopenia, post-surgical muscle atrophy, or compartment syndrome recovery

### 7.8.4 Ligamentous Injuries (e.g., MCL, ACL Sprains)

**Target** Collagenous ligament fibers

**Mechanism**
Induces ECM remodeling and fibroblast activation
Promotes neovascularization (via VEGF, HGF)
Reduces pain and inflammation

**Clinical Relevance**
Supports conservative management of partial tears
May reduce need for surgical repair in borderline cases

### 7.8.5 Bone Healing and Non-unions

**Target** Osteoblasts, osteoclasts, and periosteal microenvironment

**Mechanism**
Promotes osteogenesis (TGF-β, BMPs, VEGF, SDF-1)
Enhances bone matrix deposition and vascular perfusion
Modulates inflammatory cytokines in fracture sites

**Clinical Relevance**
Adjunct to fracture repair
May improve outcomes in stress fractures, delayed unions, and bone graft integration

### 7.8.6 Avascular Necrosis (AVN)

**Target** Ischemic bone and marrow

**Mechanism**
Induces angiogenesis and revascularization (via VEGF, HGF, bFGF)
Decreases local inflammation
Preserves viable bone structure through anti-apoptotic signaling

**Clinical Relevance**
Early-stage AVN (Ficat I–II) candidates may avoid surgery
May synergize with core decompression or orthobiologics

### 7.8.7 Enthesopathies and Insertional Tendinitis

**Target** Tendon-bone junctions

**Mechanism**
Balances inflammation at insertion sites
Enhances matrix integration and fibrocartilaginous repair
Modulates fibroblast-to-myofibroblast transitions

**Clinical Relevance**
Plantar fasciitis, gluteal tendinopathy, and tennis elbow may respond favorably
Non-invasive adjunct to loading and orthotic therapies

### 7.8.8 Fasciopathy (e.g., Plantar Fasciitis)

**Target** Dense connective tissue and fascia

**Mechanism**
Promotes collagen restructuring
Decreases neurogenic inflammation and peripheral sensitization

**Clinical Relevance**
Useful in chronic heel pain syndromes
Reduces recurrence and time to recovery

### 7.8.9 Postoperative MSK Healing Enhancement

**Target** Surgical soft tissue beds, suture sites

**Mechanism**
Enhances wound closure, reduces local inflammation
Supports ECM stability (via TSG-6, Galectin-3)
Promotes revascularization of repair zones

**Clinical Relevance**
Augmentation in rotator cuff repair, labral repair, and meniscal surgery
May reduce adhesion formation and promote functional recovery

### 7.8.10 Neuromusculoskeletal Pain Syndromes

**Target** Soft tissue–nerve interface

**Mechanism**
Downregulates pro-inflammatory mediators and pain-inducing prostaglandins (e.g., $PGE_2$)
Supports Schwann cell activity and axon repair (e.g., via miR-132, SOX2)
Enhances immune tolerance

**Clinical Relevance**

Conditions such as piriformis syndrome, thoracic outlet, or nerve entrapment with soft tissue origin

May be used adjunctively in chronic pain pathways

## 7.9 Conclusion

RCPAs offer a transformative leap in MSK regenerative care. As a cell-free, standardized, and tunable biologic platform, RCPAs bring forward the regenerative capacity of MSCs without the regulatory, immunologic, or logistical challenges of live cell therapies.

With increasing clinical interest and expanding preclinical validation, RCPAs are poised to redefine how we approach chronic degenerative conditions and acute MSK injuries. While continued research is essential, current evidence suggests that the language of regeneration can now be delivered safely, effectively, and without cells.

## Suggested Readings

Caplan AI. Mesenchymal stem cells: time to change the name! Stem Cells Transl Med. 2017;6(6):1445–51.

Galipeau J, Sensebé L. Mesenchymal stromal cells: clinical challenges and therapeutic opportunities. Cell Stem Cell. 2018;22(6):824–33.

Li Z, et al. Emerging role of exosomes in musculoskeletal diseases. Cell Commun Signal. 2021;19(1):105.

Lo Sicco C, et al. MSC-EVs mediate anti-inflammatory effects via macrophage polarization. Stem Cells Transl Med. 2017;6(3):1018–28.

Mendt M, et al. MSC-derived exosomes for clinical use. Bone Marrow Transplant. 2019;54(2):789–92.

Murphy MB, Moncivais K, Caplan AI. MSCs as responsive therapeutics. Exp Mol Med. 2013;45(11):e54.

Phinney DG, Pittenger MF. MSC-derived exosomes for cell-free therapy. Stem Cells. 2017;35(4):851–8.

Tao SC, Guo SC, Zhang CQ. Modularized extracellular vesicles for precision medicine. Adv Sci. 2018;5(2):1700449.

Vizoso FJ, et al. MSC secretome: toward cell-free therapeutic strategies in regenerative medicine. Int J Mol Sci. 2017;18(9):1852.

Yin K, Wang S, Zhao RC. Exosomes from MSCs: a new therapeutic paradigm. Biomark Res. 2019;7:8.

# Pain and the Aging Brain: Regeneration and Central Neuromodulation

# 8

Sheldon Jordan

## 8.1 Introduction

Aging remains the most significant risk factor for the development of chronic pain. As we unravel the biology of aging, the emerging concept of a central "aging clock" located in the brain opens new avenues for therapeutic intervention. Rather than viewing pain as an inevitable consequence of tissue wear, this paradigm positions pain as a measurable biomarker of neurobiological aging—one potentially modifiable through targeted neuromodulation and regenerative therapies.

This chapter explores the interplay between aging, central nervous system (CNS) regulation, and pain, with a focus on hypothalamic control of aging and emerging technologies capable of recalibrating this central clock.

The hypothalamus is a small region of the brain that plays a critical role in the following (Fig. 8.1):

- Hormonal regulation (via the pituitary gland)
- Appetite and metabolism
- Thermoregulation
- Circadian rhythms
- Stress responses
- Reproductive function

- It acts as a central control hub for many physiological processes.

S. Jordan (✉)
Regenesis Project, Santa Monica, CA, USA
e-mail: sjordan@theneuroassociates.com



R. D. Arora (ed.), *Regenerative Medicine in Pain Practice*,
https://doi.org/10.1007/978-3-032-22644-0_8

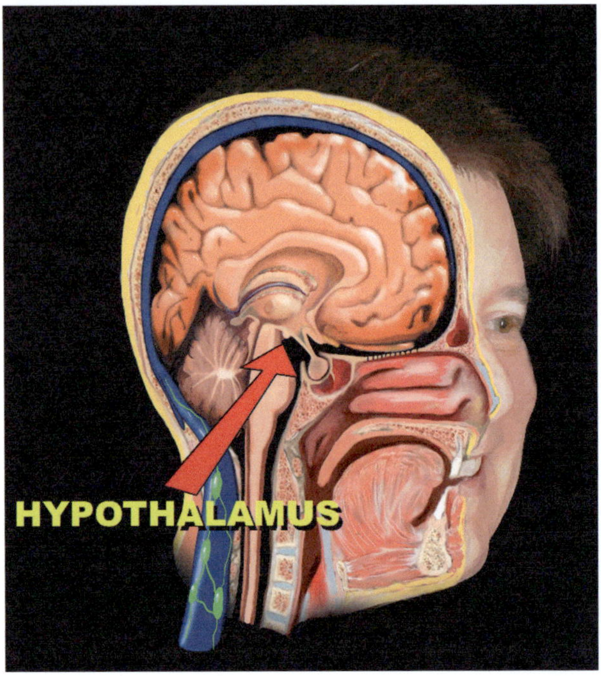


**Fig. 8.1** Hypothalamus

## 8.2 Aging and Pain: An Interconnected Timeline

Epidemiological evidence strongly supports the relationship between aging and the onset of chronic pain syndromes. Conditions such as osteoarthritis, osteoporosis, inflammatory arthritis, and axial spine pain become significantly more prevalent after the age of 40. These trends suggest not merely coincidence, but a biological entanglement—where aging and chronic pain may stem from shared central regulatory mechanisms.

## 8.3 The Central Aging Clock: Evidence and Implications

Biological timepoints—including puberty, menopause, and cognitive decline—occur with striking consistency across populations, pointing to an internal timing mechanism. In a landmark 2017 study published in *Nature*, Dr. Dongsheng Cai and colleagues demonstrated that ablation of hypothalamic stem cells in mice accelerated systemic aging, leading to hair loss, cognitive impairment, and shortened lifespan. Intriguingly, infusion of exosomes from young animals reversed these signs, restoring vitality, cognition, and sexual behavior. These findings underscore the hypothalamus—and its exosomal signaling—as a master regulator of systemic aging and potentially, pain modulation.

## 8.4 Evolutionary Framing: The Grandmother Hypothesis

The "grandmother hypothesis" offers an evolutionary explanation for regulated aging. According to this theory, elders contribute to the survival of offspring during stable times but may experience programmed decline under environmental stress to conserve resources for younger, reproductive-age individuals. This adaptive framework supports the idea of a genetically encoded, centrally regulated aging process—one that may be reversible under the right conditions.

## 8.5 Molecular Mechanisms Driving Central Aging

Age-related deterioration in the hypothalamus appears to result from multiple converging biological insults:

Melatonin decline reduces neural stem cell proliferation.
Choroid plexus calcification diminishes levels of klotho, a known anti-aging protein.

These changes disrupt neuroendocrine axes, including growth hormone, testosterone, and estrogen pathways.

They also compromise anti-inflammatory tone through the hypothalamic-pituitary-adrenal (HPA) axis and vagal cholinergic signaling, promoting systemic inflammation, sarcopenia, and chronic pain.

This cascade may explain the neuroimmune and neuroendocrine basis of chronic pain in aging.

## 8.6 Reversibility: Experimental and Clinical Prospects

Inspired by animal models, researchers are now pursuing noninvasive interventions to reset the central aging clock. One promising modality is focused ultrasound, which facilitates the delivery of exosomes and therapeutic biologics directly across the blood–brain barrier into the hypothalamus. Early trials suggest potential reversal of age-related decline and mitigation of chronic pain and muscle wasting. These findings open the door to targeted hypothalamic regeneration as a clinical strategy.

## 8.7 Neuromodulation as a Therapeutic Pathway

In parallel, neuromodulation techniques are gaining traction for their capacity to alter central pain processing. Repetitive transcranial magnetic stimulation (rTMS) applied to the primary motor cortex (M1) has produced clinically meaningful reductions in chronic neuropathic and musculoskeletal pain, with minimal side effects. Studies highlight its dual benefit: modulation of cortical pain networks and support of neuroplastic regeneration.

## 8.8 Conclusion: Resetting the Clock on Pain

Pain may not simply be a downstream product of aging—it may, in fact, be a functional output of central neurodegeneration governed by the hypothalamus. A growing body of work suggests this process can be modulated or reversed. As regenerative tools such as stem cell-derived exosomes, focused ultrasound, and neuromodulation converge, a new frontier emerges: the potential to recalibrate the aging brain and treat chronic pain at its neurological origin.

By targeting the root mechanisms of neural decline, clinicians may eventually shift from symptomatic pain relief to fundamental regeneration and lifespan extension—transforming how we approach chronic pain in aging populations.

## Selected Readings

Cai D, et al. Hypothalamic stem cells control ageing speed partly through exosomal miRNAs. Nature. 2017;548:52–7.

Hodaj H, et al. Therapeutic impact of motor cortex rTMS in chronic pain. Neurophysiol Clin. 2024;54(6):103012.

Jordan S, Zielinski M, Kortylewski M, Kuhn T, Bystritsky A Noninvasive delivery of biologicals to the brain via focused ultrasound. Focus (American Psychiatric Publishing). 2022; 20(1):64–70.

Mahdavi KD, Jordan SE, et al. Treatment of dementia with bosutinib and focused ultrasound: an open-label pilot study. J Neurodegener Disord. 2019;3(1):51–9.

# 9 Allogenic Regenerative Products in Pain Practice and Musculoskeletal Medicine

Ripu D. Arora

## 9.1 Definition and Overview

Allogenic regenerative products are ortho-biologic therapies prepared from human tissues or cells donated by another individual, rather than from the patient receiving treatment. They are intended to repair, replace, or regenerate damaged or diseased tissues in the recipient.

These products fall broadly into two categories:

**Cellular** Contain viable donor cells, such as mesenchymal stromal cells (MSCs) sourced from bone marrow, adipose tissue, umbilical cord blood or Wharton's jelly, placental tissue, or amniotic membrane.

**Acellular** Comprised of scaffolds or extracellular matrices that have been decellularized to remove donor cells while retaining the tissue structure and bioactive molecules.

The processing methods are designed to reduce immune rejection risk and disease transmission. The labs creating them must meet stringent quality and safety standards such as good manufacturing practice (GMP) and current good tissue practice (cGTP).

R. D. Arora (✉)
Arora Pain Clinic, Torrance, CA, USA



R. D. Arora (ed.), *Regenerative Medicine in Pain Practice*,
https://doi.org/10.1007/978-3-032-22644-0_9

## 9.2 Mechanisms of Action

Cellular products act primarily by:

- Secreting growth factors, cytokines, and extracellular vesicles that stimulate repair
- Modulating the immune system to reduce harmful inflammation
- Differentiating, in limited cases, into specialized tissue cells, e.g., chondrocytes and osteocytes

Acellular products work mainly by:

- Providing a structural scaffold for new tissue growth
- Retaining naturally occurring bioactive molecules that encourage cell migration, angiogenesis, and healing

## 9.3 Clinical Applications

Primary therapeutic areas include the following:

- Chronic wounds: diabetic ulcers, pressure sores, venous stasis ulcers
- Musculoskeletal (MSK) injuries and degeneration: osteoarthritis, cartilage defects, tendon or ligament injuries, meniscal tears
- Soft tissue reconstruction: following trauma, tumor excision, or surgical repair
- Certain inflammatory conditions: perianal fistulas in Crohn's disease and other selected autoimmune pathologies

Common orthopedic applications:

- Intra-articular injections for knee osteoarthritis and cartilage repair
- Augmentation of tendon and ligament repair surgeries
- Treatment of osteochondral lesions in the ankle, shoulder, or elbow
- Reconstruction of bone defects, including nonunion and avascular necrosis

## 9.4 Patient Selection

Before initiating treatment with allogenic regenerative products, a thorough assessment should be performed to ensure safety and optimize outcomes. This should include the following:

- Comprehensive review of medical history and assessment of comorbid conditions.
- Detailed physical examination of the affected area

- Relevant laboratory testing and imaging studies appropriate to the condition and planned intervention
- Immunologic assessment in patients with known risk factors for graft rejection or adverse immune responses

### 9.4.1 Absolute Contraindications

Treatment should not be performed in the presence of active systemic or local infection.

Known allergy or hypersensitivity to any product components.

Malignancy located at or near the intended treatment site.

History of severe allergies or immune reaction to donor-derived products.

Use of products from inadequately screened donors.

### 9.4.2 Relative Contraindications

Caution is advised and risk–benefit should be carefully considered in:

- Immunosuppressed or immunodeficient individuals
- Pregnant or breastfeeding patients
- Patients with uncontrolled autoimmune disease
- Areas of poor local vascularity where graft incorporation may be compromised

## 9.5 Administration and Monitoring

**Delivery Methods**

Injectable formulations for direct placement into joints, tendons, or wound beds

Surgical implantation of grafts, patches, or particulate material

**Monitoring Protocols**

Immediate observation post-procedure for allergic or infusion reactions

Short-term follow-up for signs of infection, inflammation, or immune response

Long-term surveillance for treatment durability, delayed rejection, and functional recovery

**Documentation**

Should include product identity, processing method, delivery technique, patient condition, and all observed outcomes

## 9.6 Safety and Risk Profile

**Common Mild Effects**
Temporary pain, swelling, or stiffness at the treatment site

**Rare but Serious Risks**
Infectious disease transmission (extremely rare with proper screening)
Immune-mediated tissue rejection (more likely with viable cellular products)
Graft failure or mechanical breakdown in structural applications
Theoretical risk of tumor formation with certain cell-based products (low with adult MSCs)

Risks are lowest with acellular or decellularized products and highest with viable, poorly processed grafts.

### 9.6.1 Regulatory Considerations (US)

The FDA regulates allogenic regenerative products under the HCT/P framework:

Section 351 Products: More than minimally manipulated or nonhomologous use; regulated as biologics or drugs; require IND (investigational new drug application) for clinical use and BLA (biologics license application) for marketing.
Section 361 Products: Minimally manipulated and homologous use; require FDA registration and communicable disease prevention compliance; no premarket approval.

**Common Off-Label MSK Applications**
- Intra-articular injections for knee osteoarthritis
- Repair of focal cartilage defects
- Surgical augmentation for tendon, ligament, and meniscus repair
- Treatment of osteochondral lesions in the ankle and shoulder

These applications are investigational and generally lack FDA approval for MSK indications.

**Comparative Use—Allogenic Versus Autologous Orthobiologics**
*Allogenic products may be preferred when:*
Autologous tissue harvest is unsafe or impractical
Rapid "off-the-shelf" availability is necessary
Pediatric or adolescent patients require treatment (avoid donor site morbidity)
Large graft volumes or specialized tissue types are required
*Autologous products may be preferred when*:

Immune compatibility is a concern
Regulatory barriers to allogenic use limit access
The patient's own tissue can be harvested without significant morbidity

**Summary**
This framework provides a practical approach for integrating allogenic regenerative products into MSK care. It emphasizes safe administration, vigilant monitoring, a clear understanding of regulatory boundaries, recognition of off-label use scenarios, and an informed comparison with autologous alternatives to guide product selection.

## 9.7 Allogenic Regenerative Products in Musculoskeletal Medicine—Procedural Applications and Evidence (Table 9.1)

### 9.7.1 Knee Osteoarthritis (OA)

**Rationale**
Knee OA is the most common target for intra-articular allogenic regenerative therapies. These products aim to reduce pain, improve joint function, and potentially slow cartilage degeneration through anti-inflammatory and anabolic signaling.

**Common Allogenic Products**
Umbilical cord–derived MSCs
Amniotic membrane particulate or fluid products
Placenta-derived MSC suspensions
Decellularized extracellular matrix injectates

**Procedure—Intra-Articular Injection**
Preparation: Patient positioned supine with the knee extended; aseptic skin preparation and draping.
Landmark Identification: Superolateral or anterolateral approach to the suprapatellar pouch is preferred.
Injection: Confirm intra-articular placement by aspirating synovial fluid or using ultrasound guidance. Deliver 1–4 mL of product via a 21–25G needle.
Post-Procedure: Limit weight-bearing for 24–48 h; avoid NSAIDs (nonsteroidal anti-inflammatory drugs) for the first 72 h to preserve biological activity.

**Evidence Summary**
Meta-analyses show clinically significant pain and function improvements for up to 12 months, with some extending to 24 months.
Benefits are comparable to autologous bone marrow aspirate concentrate (BMAC) and platelet-rich plasma (PRP) in the short- to mid-term.
Structural cartilage regeneration remains unconfirmed, with variable imaging findings.

**Table 9.1** Allogenic regenerative applications in MSK disorders

| Condition | Common products | Delivery method | Typical benefit window | Evidence insights | Evidence grade |
|---|---|---|---|---|---|
| Knee OA | UC-MSC, amniotic injectates | Intra-articular | 6–24 months | Pain/function gains; comparable to PRP/BMAC | II |
| Rotator cuff tear | Dermal allograft, amniotic patch | Arthroscopic augmentation | 6–12 months | Lower re-tear rates, modest functional improvement | II |
| Talus OCD | Osteochondral allograft | Open/ arthroscopic implantation | 2–5+ years | High graft survival, good function | II |
| Talus OCD | Particulated juvenile cartilage | Open/ arthroscopic implantation | 1–3 years | Early gains; limited long-term data | III |
| Meniscal loss | Meniscal allograft | Arthroscopic transplant | 5–10 years | Functional gain, slower OA progression | II |
| Bone defect | Structural allograft, DBM | Open grafting | Variable | Union rates comparable to autograft in select settings | II |
| Bone defect | Cellular allograft | Open grafting | Variable | Early promise; lacks high-quality trials | III |

### 9.7.2 Rotator Cuff Repair Augmentation

**Rationale**

High re-tear rates after rotator cuff repair have driven interest in biologic augmentation. Allogenic patches and extracellular matrix (ECM) scaffolds can improve tendon-bone healing by providing structural support and bioactive materials.

**Common Allogenic Products**

- Decellularized dermal allografts
- Amniotic membrane patches
- Collagen-rich ECM scaffolds

**Procedure—Surgical Augmentation**

Arthroscopic Repair: Standard tendon mobilization and fixation using suture anchors.

Graft Preparation: Hydrate the matrix as per manufacturer protocol; trim to match the tendon footprint.

Patch Placement: Secure over the repair site with sutures or anchors; ensure tension-free placement.

Rehabilitation: Sling immobilization for 4–6 weeks; gradual transition from passive to active range of motion.

**Evidence Summary**

Observational pooled data indicate lower re-tear rates at 6–12 months compared to repair alone.

Functional improvements are modest but clinically significant.

Greatest benefit is observed in large or massive tears.

### 9.7.3 Osteochondral Lesions of the Talus

**Rationale**

These lesions are challenging due to limited intrinsic healing capacity. Allogenic osteochondral grafts and particulated juvenile cartilage provide mature hyaline cartilage structure and viable chondrocytes.

**Common Allogenic Products**

Fresh osteochondral allografts

Particulated juvenile cartilage allograft chips

**Procedure—Open or Arthroscopic Implantation**

Defect Debridement: Remove unstable cartilage and sclerotic bone.

Graft Sizing: Harvest matched plugs for fresh allografts; measure defect size for particulated cartilage.

Graft Insertion: Press-fit osteochondral plugs flush with surrounding cartilage. For particulated cartilage, fill defect and secure with fibrin glue.

Postoperative Protocol: Non-weight-bearing for 6–8 weeks, then gradual load progression.

**Evidence Summary**

Fresh allografts demonstrate high defect filling and good functional outcomes, with >80% survival at 5 years.

Particulated juvenile cartilage provides early gains, though long-term durability data are limited.

### 9.7.4 Meniscal Allograft Transplantation

**Rationale**

Loss of meniscal tissue increases contact pressures and accelerates joint degeneration. Meniscal transplantation restores load distribution and can delay osteoarthritic progression.

**Procedure Highlights**

Arthroscopic or mini-open approach
Bone plug or bone bridge fixation to recreate anatomical attachment
Peripheral fixation with centralization sutures
Protected weight-bearing for 6 weeks postoperatively

**Evidence Summary**

Significant improvements in knee function scores.
Return-to-sport rates between 60% and 80%.
Radiographic progression of arthritis is slowed but not completely prevented.

### 9.7.5 Bone Defects and Nonunion

**Rationale**

Critical-sized bone defects and atrophic nonunions often require grafting for structural stability and osteogenesis. Allogenic bone grafts offer structural support, and cellular allografts may add biological activity.

**Common Allogenic Products**

Fresh-frozen cortical or cancellous bone
Demineralized bone matrix (DBM) with or without added cells

**Procedure—Grafting**

Debridement: Remove fibrous tissue and necrotic bone to healthy margins.
Graft Placement: Press-fit or pack graft material into the defect.
Stabilization: Use plate, nail, or external fixation as indicated.

**Evidence Summary**

Structural allografts achieve union rates comparable to autografts in select cases, with slower incorporation.
Cellular allografts are promising but lack robust high-quality comparative data.

### 9.7.6 Monitoring and Outcome Assessment (Cross-Application)

Short-term: Monitor for local reaction, infection, and early pain response.
Mid-term: Evaluate functional scores (WOMAC, IKDC, ASES, FAOS), return-to-activity metrics.
Long-term: Imaging to assess graft integrity, survival rates, and delayed complications.

**Evidence Grade Definitions**
- *I*—Multiple high-quality randomized controlled trials (RCTs) or meta-analysis of RCTs
- *II*—Single high-quality RCT or meta-analysis of lower-level studies
- *III*—Cohort studies, case-control studies, or large case series
- *IV*—Expert opinion, small case series, or preclinical data only

## 9.8 Cord Blood (Umbilical)–Derived Cellular Therapies

Cord blood (CB) has become an important source of cellular therapies due to its unique biological composition. Compared with adult peripheral blood (PB), CB contains a higher percentage of natural killer (NK) cells and a rich pool of hematopoietic stem cells (HSCs). These cells are more naïve, exhibit lower immunogenicity, and possess greater proliferation potential, making CB a highly attractive resource for regenerative and immunotherapeutic applications (Fig. 9.1).

**HSCs:**
- Widely used in hematopoietic stem cell transplantation (HCT).
- Provide a renewable source for induced pluripotent stem cells (iPSCs).
- Play a central role in regenerative medicine strategies.

**T Cells:**
- Can be engineered into allogeneic chimeric antigen receptor cells (CAR T cells) for cancer immunotherapy.
- Serve as a source for regulatory T cells (Tregs) and CAR T-regs to promote immune tolerance.
- Expanded to generate virus-specific T cells (VSTs) for treatment of viral infections.

**NK Cells:**
- Readily available from CB for unmodified NK cell infusion.
- Can be modified to form CAR NK cells with potent antitumor effects.
- May be pre-activated or combined with NK cell engagers for enhanced therapeutic outcomes.

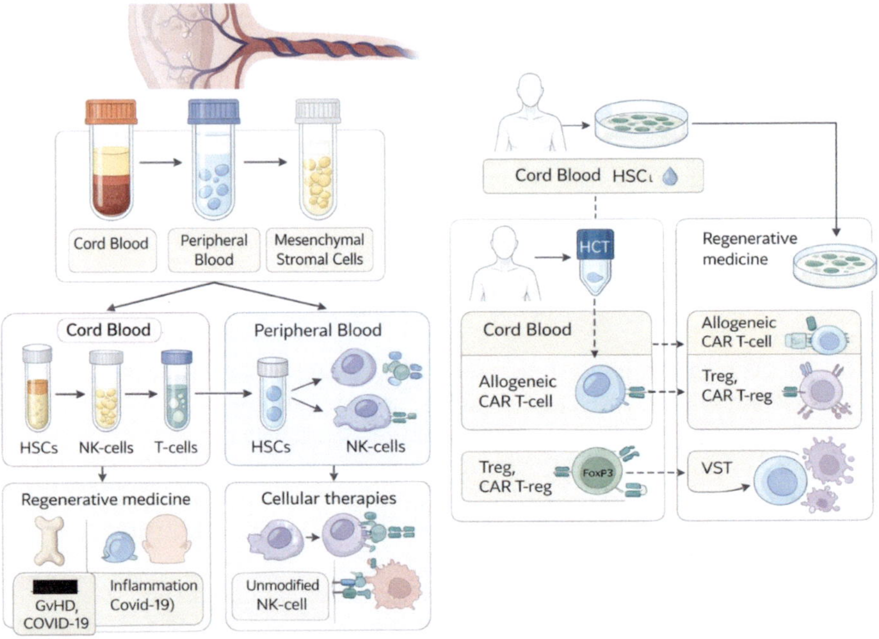


**Fig. 9.1** Overview of cord blood–derived therapies. The diagram illustrates the spectrum of CB-derived products and their applications. CB contains HSCs, NK cells, and T cells that can be directed toward transplantation, regenerative medicine, or advanced immunotherapies. Additionally, Wharton's jelly provides MSCs with regenerative and immunomodulatory potential. Collectively, these components make CB a versatile source for treating hematologic, autoimmune, inflammatory, and degenerative conditions

**Wharton's Jelly–Derived MSCs:**

- Possess regenerative, immunomodulatory, and anti-inflammatory properties.
- Useful in regenerative medicine and tissue engineering.
- Show promise in autoimmune and inflammatory diseases.

## 9.9 CB Products Versus Wharton's Jelly in Allogenic MSK Therapies

In the context of allogenic regenerative therapies for MSK disorders, CB and Wharton's jelly represent two distinct sources within the umbilical cord, each with unique biological characteristics and clinical implications.

CB products are obtained from the blood contained within the umbilical cord and are naturally rich in HSCs. They also contain MSCs, but at relatively low concentrations compared to other cord compartments. These MSCs have a distinct profile, with some evidence suggesting lower proliferative capacity and reduced adipogenic differentiation potential compared to MSCs from Wharton's jelly. CB products have been explored for regenerative and immunomodulatory applications, but their limited MSC yield often requires larger collection volumes and more complex processing to achieve therapeutic cell doses.

Wharton's jelly is the gelatinous connective tissue that surrounds the umbilical vessels. It is a highly enriched source of MSCs, providing greater cell numbers, higher purity, and superior proliferative capacity than CB. Wharton's jelly–derived MSCs demonstrate enhanced stemness, stronger chondrogenic and osteogenic differentiation potential, and robust immunomodulatory effects. They also have low immunogenicity, making them attractive for allogenic use. Clinical studies in MSK disorders, including knee OA, have reported improvements in pain, function, and imaging findings after intra-articular injections of Wharton's jelly MSCs, with some evidence of increased cartilage thickness and favorable changes in synovial biomarkers over the course of a year.

*Clinical considerations when choosing between the two sources include the following*:

*Cellular yield and quality*—Wharton's jelly provides significantly higher MSC yields with greater proliferation and shorter culture times, while CB MSCs are less abundant and often mixed with non-stem cell components.

*Differentiation and regenerative potential*—Wharton's jelly MSCs have superior capacity for muscle, bone, and cartilage differentiation, and a beneficial secretome profile that supports tissue repair and modulates inflammation in degenerative conditions.

*Clinical evidence*—More consistent positive outcomes have been reported for Wharton's jelly MSCs in MSK disorders, whereas data for CB MSCs are more variable and less abundant.

*Practical, ethical, and regulatory aspects*—Wharton's jelly is easier to process with minimal manipulation, enabling more standardized large-scale production. CB banking and processing involve greater logistical complexity, higher cost, and potential ethical considerations. Regulatory trends increasingly favor sources with reproducible quality and safety profiles.

## 9.10 Summary

Wharton's jelly–derived products generally offer advantages over CB products for MSK regenerative medicine, including higher MSC content, superior regenerative potential, stronger supporting clinical data, and greater ease of processing and standardization. Both remain investigational, and direct high-quality comparative clinical trials are needed to fully establish their optimal roles (Table 9.2).

**Table 9.2** Comparison of Wharton's Jelly and CB in MSK allogenic therapies

| Feature | Wharton's Jelly | Umbilical cord blood (CB) |
|---|---|---|
| Tissue source | Gelatinous connective tissue surrounding umbilical vessels | Blood within the umbilical cord |
| Primary stem cell type | MSCs | HSCs with a smaller MSC population |
| MSC yield | High; abundant and easy to isolate | Low; requires large volume collection and complex isolation |
| Proliferation potential | High; faster expansion and lower senescence | Lower proliferation; longer culture times |
| Differentiation potential | Strong chondrogenic, osteogenic, and myogenic capacity | Limited chondrogenic/osteogenic capacity compared to Wharton's Jelly |
| Immunomodulatory properties | Robust; low immunogenicity and strong anti-inflammatory profile | Present, but generally less pronounced |
| Clinical evidence in MSK disorders | More consistent results; improvements in pain, function, cartilage thickness | Limited and variable; fewer controlled studies |
| Processing & standardization | Easier to standardize; minimal manipulation possible | More complex logistics; higher variability between samples |
| Regulatory considerations | Favorable for large-scale production; well-suited for homologous use frameworks | More regulatory hurdles; potential ethical and legal issues |
| Overall MSK regenerative potential | High; preferred for many investigational applications | Moderate; potential niche roles but less scalable |

## 9.11 Future of Allogenic Regenerative Medicine in MSK Disorders (US Perspective)

The future of regenerative medicine in the United States especially in the treatment of MSK disorders using allogenic regenerative products is rapidly evolving. Innovation in biologic materials, increased clinical interest, and ongoing regulatory refinement are shaping the development and clinical integration of these therapies.

Allogenic products, including perinatal tissue–derived MSCs and amniotic membrane–based formulations, are being explored extensively due to their off-the-shelf availability and their applicability in patients for whom autologous tissue harvest is contraindicated or impractical. These products eliminate the need for donor site morbidity and offer immediate accessibility, which is especially beneficial for elderly individuals, immunocompromised patients, or those with limited regenerative potential.

Early clinical studies in indications such as knee OA, focal cartilage defects, tendon pathology, and bone regeneration have demonstrated encouraging safety profiles and preliminary functional improvements. However, high-quality RCTs with long-term follow-up remain limited. The translation of these promising findings into routine clinical practice will require stronger evidence demonstrating consistent, reproducible outcomes over time.

From a regulatory standpoint, allogenic injectable products derived from perinatal tissue remain largely unapproved for MSK indications in the United States. Federal agencies have clarified that many of these products do not meet criteria for homologous use or minimal manipulation and therefore fall under regulatory pathways that require formal approval before clinical use. This includes IND applications and BLA. Agencies continue to scrutinize manufacturing, labeling, and marketing practices to ensure patient safety and scientific integrity.

Looking forward, advances in gene-edited stem cells, 3D bioprinting, nanotechnology-assisted delivery systems, and combination therapies incorporating scaffolds, growth factors, and cells may dramatically enhance therapeutic capabilities. These evolving technologies will allow for the tailoring of biologic interventions to the patient's pathology and biology, potentially ushering in a new era of personalized MSK regenerative care.

However, the successful future of allogenic regenerative medicine depends on three foundational pillars:

**Standardization of Preparation**
Harmonized protocols and quality controls are essential to ensure product consistency, reproducibility, and safety.

**Robust Clinical Evidence**
Widespread adoption will require high-level clinical trials demonstrating clear superiority or non-inferiority to existing treatments, along with long-term durability of outcomes.

**Ethical and Transparent Communication**
Clinicians and stakeholders must commit to responsible dissemination of benefits and risks, aligning patient expectations with available evidence, and avoiding premature marketing of investigational products.

As regulatory clarity improves and the clinical evidence base strengthens, allogenic regenerative products may become a cornerstone in the multidisciplinary treatment of MSK pathology, especially for patients with limited options in traditional surgical and conservative care paradigms.

## 9.12 Conclusion

Allogenic regenerative products are biologic therapies derived from donor human tissues or cells and are increasingly used in MSK medicine to repair, replace, or regenerate damaged structures. These products may be cellular, such as MSCs from bone marrow, adipose, or perinatal sources, or acellular, such as decellularized extracellular matrices and processed tissue allografts. Their mechanisms include paracrine signaling, immunomodulation, and provision of structural scaffolds. Current applications in orthopedics and sports medicine include intra-articular injections for OA, biologic augmentation of tendon and ligament repairs, osteochondral defect reconstruction, meniscal allograft transplantation, and bone defect filling. While meta-analyses support symptom improvement and functional gains for several indications, high-level evidence for structural regeneration remains limited, and most uses are off label under current regulatory frameworks. Proper patient selection, adherence to manufacturing and handling standards, and rigorous post-procedure monitoring are essential to optimize outcomes and minimize risks such as infection, immune reaction, or graft failure. Regulatory classification by the U.S. Food and Drug Administration determines permissible clinical use, with most orthopedic indications for allogenic injectables falling under investigational oversight. Future advances in cell processing, tissue engineering, and combined biologic strategies hold promise, but widespread adoption depends on long-term safety data, standardization, and high-quality randomized trials.

**Key Points**

Allogenic regenerative products are derived from donor human tissues or cells and include both cellular and acellular forms.

Used in MSK medicine for OA, tendon and ligament repair augmentation, osteochondral lesion reconstruction, meniscal allograft transplantation, and bone defect filling.

Most orthopedic uses are off label under U.S. FDA regulations; strongest evidence supports symptom and function improvement.

Optimal outcomes require patient selection, safety and handling protocols, and structured post-procedure monitoring.

Future growth depends on standardization, long-term safety data, and high-quality trials.

## Suggested Readings

Caplan AI. Mesenchymal stem cells: biology, mechanisms, and clinical applications.

Migliorini F. Allogenic vs. autologous bone grafts for orthopedic reconstruction: a systematic review and meta-analysis.

Orthopedic Research Society. Clinical guidelines on the use of orthobiologics in musculoskeletal disorders.

Rosso F. Meniscal allograft transplantation: outcomes and long-term survival.

U.S. Food and Drug Administration. Regulatory considerations for human cells, tissues, and cellular and tissue-based products.

Vangsness CT Jr. Allogenic mesenchymal stem cells for cartilage and meniscus regeneration.

# Integrating Regenerative Medicine Within Pain Management Practice

# 10

Ripu D. Arora

Chronic pain is a complex, multifactorial condition that often necessitates a multi-modal treatment strategy. Traditional approaches have provided symptomatic relief, but emerging modalities such as regenerative medicine offer disease-modifying potential by addressing the underlying tissue pathology.

## 10.1 Conventional Pain Management Modalities

Conventional Pain Management Modalities have Their own shortcomings (Table 10.1)

The therapeutic landscape includes:

### 10.1.1 Medication/Opioids

Widely used for pain suppression.

Risks include dependence, tolerance, and systemic side effects.

Best suited for short-term or palliative care

### 10.1.2 Physical Therapy

Enhances mobility and strengthens supportive musculature.

Addresses biomechanical contributors to pain.

Optimal when combined with other therapies

R. D. Arora (✉)
Arora Pain Clinic, Torrance, CA, USA



R. D. Arora (ed.), *Regenerative Medicine in Pain Practice*,
https://doi.org/10.1007/978-3-032-22644-0_10

**Table 10.1** Stem cells vs. traditional treatments

| Aspect | Stem cell therapy | Traditional surgery |
|---|---|---|
| Approach | Natural healing by regenerating tissues | Structural repair, often more definitive for severe injuries |
| Effectiveness | Often long-lasting with significant pain relief and improved joint function for years | Effective for severe damage that stem cells may not fix |
| Invasiveness | Less invasive | More invasive |
| Recovery and risks | Lower risk of complications | Longer recovery times; higher risk of complications (e.g., infections, blood clots, joint stiffness) |
| Longevity of results | Sustained benefits reported | Artificial joints may wear out, requiring revision surgery |

### 10.1.3 Steroid Injections

Anti-inflammatory relief for localized conditions (e.g., joint, spine).

Benefits are temporary and repeated use may weaken tissue integrity.

### 10.1.4 Interventional Procedures

Includes nerve blocks, facet injections, and radiofrequency ablation, PNS & SCS (Peripheral Nerve Stimulation & Spinal Cord Stimulation) neuromodulation techniques that interfere with pain signal transmission.

Effective in neuropathic and refractory pain cases.

Typically, these procedures are targeted and minimally invasive but are primarily symptom-focused.

### 10.1.5 Surgery

Reserved for structural abnormalities or failed conservative care.

High-risk and often associated with variable outcomes in chronic pain.

## 10.2 Benefits of Adding Regenerative Therapy in Pain Practice

Regenerative medicine, particularly stem cell-based therapies, is transforming the landscape of pain management. Its advantages extend beyond symptom control, offering comprehensive improvements in patient outcomes and healthcare efficiency including the following.

### 10.2.1 Reduced Medication Usage and Costs

One of the most significant advantages of regenerative therapy is its potential to substantially reduce the reliance on pain medications, including opioids and anti-inflammatories. As pain levels decrease and joint function improves, patients often report reduced need for long-term pharmacological support, lowering both the financial burden and the risk of medication-related side effects and dependency.

### 10.2.2 Cost Savings from Reduced Injection Requirements

Conventional treatments for chronic pain such as corticosteroid or hyaluronic acid injections often require repeated administration. Regenerative therapies may offer a longer lasting solution, reducing the frequency and need for these additional interventions, which results in lower cumulative healthcare costs over time.

### 10.2.3 Avoidance of Surgery: Savings in Pain and Money

For many patients, regenerative medicine offers a viable alternative to orthopedic or spinal surgeries. Avoiding surgery not only prevents the physical and emotional toll of invasive procedures but also eliminates associated expenses such as hospitalization, anesthesia, and postoperative rehabilitation. This dual benefit of pain relief and financial savings makes regenerative therapy particularly attractive.

### 10.2.4 Significant Pain Reduction or Elimination

Many patients experience a dramatic decrease in chronic pain symptoms following stem cell therapy. In some cases, pain is eliminated. This improvement is often attributed to the regenerative potential of stem cells, which reduce inflammation, repair damaged tissues, and restore joint health at a cellular level.

### 10.2.5 Marked Improvement in Functionality

Beyond pain control, regenerative medicine helps restore physical function. Patients frequently report improved mobility, increased range of motion, and joint stability, enabling patients to return to their daily activities including work and hobbies that were previously limited or impossible due to chronic pain.

### 10.2.6 Challenging the Traditional Medical Model

Regenerative therapy represents a fundamental shift away from the conventional "replace and suppress" model of medicine. Instead of masking symptoms or replacing damaged parts, this approach focuses on biological restoration and healing. It disrupts traditional paradigms and encourages a shift toward curative and minimally invasive therapies.

### 10.2.7 Cutting-Edge Innovation in Clinical Care

The field of regenerative medicine sits at the intersection of biotechnology, cellular biology, and personalized medicine. It exemplifies modern innovation in healthcare, offering patients access to advanced therapies grounded in scientific research and precision medicine. Its evolving nature ensures ongoing improvements and new applications.

### 10.2.8 Unique Ability to Induce Regeneration

Most importantly, regenerative therapy is the only current clinical approach that actively induces tissue regeneration. Unlike other modalities that replace or support failing tissues, stem cells can stimulate the body's own repair mechanisms, leading to true biological healing. This makes regenerative therapy a cornerstone in the future of pain medicine.

### 10.2.9 Regenerative Medicine: A Paradigm Shift

Regenerative medicine aims to restore, replace, or regenerate damaged tissues rather than merely suppressing symptoms. Treatment options include the use of the following:

- Platelet-rich plasma (PRP).
- Bone marrow aspirate concentrate (BMAC).
- Adipose-derived stem cells.
- Exosome therapy.

These biologics modulate inflammation, promote tissue healing, and improve functional recovery especially in degenerative joint disease, tendon pathology, and neuropathic injuries.

## 10.3 Conclusion: The Clinical Promise of Regenerative Medicine in Pain Practice

Regenerative medicine represents a transformative advancement in pain management, offering a biologically sound, patient-centered approach to tissue healing and inflammation control. By harnessing the body's own repair mechanisms, regenerative therapies offer not only symptomatic relief but also the potential for long-term functional restoration creating a paradigm shift from traditional treatments focused primarily on symptom suppression.

### 10.3.1 A Safe, Autologous Approach

One of the foremost advantages of regenerative therapy is its autologous nature which means it is derived from the patient's own tissues. This eliminates the risk of immunogenic reactions or disease transmission and provides a biologically compatible reservoir of therapeutic agents, including growth factors, cytokines, and anti-inflammatory mediators. These components promote anabolic remodeling of damaged tissue and modulate inflammation, laying the foundation for true recovery rather than temporary relief.

### 10.3.2 Diverse Sources and Mechanisms

Modern regenerative protocols utilize a wide array of autologous products such as PRP, concentrated plasma, autologous serum, and platelet lysates. These preparations are rich in bioactive molecules like Interleukin-1 Receptor Antagonist Protein (IRAP) and Alpha-2-Macroglobulin (A2M), which are known to counteract inflammatory pathways and protect cartilage from degeneration. The diversity of formulations allows clinicians to tailor treatment based on the clinical condition, targeted tissue, and desired biological response.

### 10.3.3 Low-Risk Profile and Retained Options

Compared to invasive surgical procedures or chronic pharmacologic regimens involving steroids or opioids, regenerative therapies offer a low-risk alternative. If a patient does not experience adequate benefit, they are no worse off biologically than before the procedure—unlike surgery, which is irreversible. Importantly, all other treatment options remain viable, giving both the clinician and patient flexibility in managing care without burning any bridges.

### 10.3.4 Comparable Safety in Spinal Applications

Emerging evidence and clinical experience indicate that the biological safety of regenerative products is comparable to procedures already considered standard, such as epidural blood patches for spinal CSF leaks. This expands the applicability of regenerative therapy into the spinal and epidural realms, reinforcing its relevance in complex pain syndromes, particularly in patients for whom steroids or surgery are contraindicated.

### 10.3.5 Practical Delivery and Familiar Techniques

Regenerative products can be administered using standard interventional pain techniques, such as ultrasound-guided or fluoroscopy-assisted injections. This makes integration into practice seamless for pain physicians who are already proficient in such procedures, requiring only minimal additional training.

### 10.3.6 Customizability and Patient-Specific Optimization

One of the most compelling features of regenerative therapy is the ability to customize concentrations and components. Factors such as centrifugation speed, plasma volume, and the inclusion or exclusion of leukocytes can be adjusted based on the pathology and patient response. This level of biological precision is unmatched by most pharmacological approaches and positions regenerative medicine at the forefront of personalized care.

### 10.3.7 Conclusion

Regenerative medicine is not just a novel intervention; it is a revolutionary therapy reifying the body's own intrinsic healing potential. As safety profiles improve, and outcomes data amass, we will see advances in regulations that position regenerative therapies as the mainstay in the management of musculoskeletal and neuropathic pain. The journey from symptomatic relief to biological restoration is underway, and regenerative medicine is at the helm of that evolution.

# Regulatory Considerations in Regenerative Medicine

# 11

Ripu D. Arora

## 11.1 Introduction

In the United States, the use and marketing of regenerative medicine products, particularly those involving human cells, tissues, and cellular or tissue-based products (HCT/Ps), are governed by federal regulations under 21 CFR Part 1271. These rules are designed to ensure patient safety while fostering innovation in this rapidly evolving field.

21 CFR 1271 grants the U.S. Food and Drug Administration (FDA) the authority to oversee the development and clinical use of HCT/Ps. The regulation primarily aims to prevent the transmission of communicable diseases and to ensure proper handling and labeling of these products.

## 11.2 Categories of Biologic Products: Class 351 vs. Class 361 (Table 11.1)

Under FDA guidelines, applicable biologics are classified into two major categories, each with distinct regulatory pathways:

### 11.2.1 Class 351 Products

These are considered biologic drugs. As such, they must undergo the full FDA approval process, including extensive clinical trials, safety and efficacy evaluations, and a Biologics License Application (BLA). Examples include expanded or cultured stem cell products or any HCT/Ps that are more than minimally manipulated or intended for non-homologous use.

R. D. Arora (✉)
Arora Pain Clinic, Torrance, CA, USA



R. D. Arora (ed.), *Regenerative Medicine in Pain Practice*,
https://doi.org/10.1007/978-3-032-22644-0_11

**Table 11.1** Comparison of class 351 and class 361 products

| Criteria | Class 351 products | Class 361 products |
|---|---|---|
| Regulatory classification | Biologic Drug | Human Cell and Tissue Product (HCT/P) |
| FDA approval required | Yes, requires BLA and FDA approval | No, if criteria in 21 CFR 1271.10 are met |
| Definition | More than minimally manipulated or non-homologous use | Minimally manipulated and intended for homologous use |
| Level of manipulation | More than minimal manipulation | Minimal manipulation only |
| Type of use | Non-homologous (used for a different function than in donor) | Homologous (used for same function as in donor) |
| Examples | Expanded stem cell cultures, gene-edited cells | PRP (Platelet Rich Plasma), bone marrow aspirate, adipose tissue (minimally processed) |
| Oversight | Strict FDA oversight through CDER (Center for Drug Evaluation and Research) or CBER (Center for Biologics Evaluation and Research) | Less stringent oversight under 21 CFR 1271 |
| Clinical trials needed | Yes, clinical trials and data submission required | No, clinical trials not required unless conditions change |

### 11.2.2 Class 361 Products

These are not considered drugs and therefore do not require premarket FDA approval, as long as they meet the specific criteria outlined in 21 CFR 1271.10. These criteria include requirements for minimal manipulation, homologous use, and lack of systemic effect unless intended for autologous use or for a close relative.

This bifurcation is essential because it allows the use of certain regenerative therapies under physician supervision without the need for lengthy regulatory approval, provided they adhere to defined limitations.

## 11.3 2017 CBER Guidance Document: Clarifying FDA Criteria

To provide greater clarity to clinicians and industry stakeholders, the FDA's CBER released a Guidance Document in 2017. This document outlined key regulatory concepts that determine whether a product is subject to full drug approval.

The two core principles defined were as follows:

### 11.3.1 Minimal Manipulation

This means that the biological characteristics, functions, or structural properties of the cells or tissues are not altered beyond what is necessary for their intended use.

### 11.3.2 Homologous Use

This requires that the HCT/P be used to perform the same basic function in the recipient as it does in the donor. For instance, using stem cells derived from adipose tissue to repair or regenerate musculoskeletal tissues is not considered homologous use unless clearly justified.

These concepts help providers and manufacturers assess whether their interventions fall within regulatory exemptions or if they require formal FDA clearance.

## 11.4 Exceptions to 21 CFR 1271

The Case of PRP and Autologous Blood Products

An important exception to the strict regulatory oversight outlined above involves autologous blood products including PRP. When these products are minimally manipulated and used for homologous purposes, they are not subject to FDA regulation as HCT/Ps under the 21 CFR 1271 framework.

Key Points on PRP Regulation

### 11.4.1 PRP Is Not Regulated as a Biologic

Because PRP is derived from the patient's own blood and involves only minimal processing (e.g., centrifugation), it falls outside the definition of a drug or biologic product when used appropriately.

### 11.4.2 PRP Is Not Classified as a Drug

No drug labeling or FDA marketing approval is required when PRP is prepared and administered in accordance with standard medical practices.

### 11.4.3 Use Under the Practice of Medicine

Physicians are permitted to use PRP under the scope of their professional discretion, often referred to as the "practice of medicine." This autonomy allows tailored treatments to meet individual patient needs without federal regulatory interference—so long as the use remains compliant with established safety guidelines.

## 11.5 Implications for Clinical Practice

Understanding these regulatory nuances is essential for clinicians engaged in regenerative therapies. While innovation continues to expand possibilities, providers must remain vigilant to ensure compliance with federal rules. Misclassification or off-label use of HCT/Ps without proper authorization can lead to significant legal and ethical consequences.

By adhering to the criteria for minimal manipulation and homologous use and by recognizing exceptions such as PRP, clinicians can confidently integrate regenerative techniques into pain management practices, advancing care while staying within regulatory bounds.

## Suggested Readings

Deans RJ, Rasko JE. Cellular therapies: regulatory and commercialization challenges. Nat Rev Drug Discov. 2021;20:415–6.

FDA21 CFR Part 1271 – Human cells, tissues, and cellular and tissue-based products. 2017. Retrieved from https://www.ecfr.gov/current/title-21/part-1271

Rybicki BA. Regulatory overview of regenerative medicine in the United States. J Transl Med. 2017;15(1):195.

U.S. Food and Drug Administration. Regulatory considerations for human cells, tissues, and cellular and tissue-based products: minimal manipulation and homologous use. 2020. Retrieved from https://www.fda.gov/media/109176/download

# Regenerative Medicine Marketing and Business Development

12

Ripu D. Arora

## 12.1 Introduction

Regenerative medicine holds the promise of revolutionizing the way we approach chronic pain and musculoskeletal conditions. By leveraging the body's own healing potential through treatments like platelet-rich plasma (PRP), bone marrow aspirate, and other cell-based therapies, this emerging field provides non-surgical, personalized solutions for conditions that were previously difficult to manage. Despite its growing clinical potential, regenerative medicine remains underutilized. Barriers such as low public awareness, regulatory gray zones, and inconsistent practice marketing continue to hinder its widespread adoption. This chapter explores a step-by-step, experience-driven approach to marketing and growing a regenerative medicine practice, anchored in ethics, compliance, and patient education.

## 12.2 The Need for Marketing in Regenerative Medicine

Regenerative therapies offer innovative alternatives, yet most patients and even many physicians are unaware of these options or are uncertain about their efficacy. Because of this, proactive marketing is not optional, it is essential. Unlike traditional specialties where referral pipelines are well-established, regenerative medicine must often reach patients directly.

R. D. Arora (✉)
Arora Pain Clinic, Torrance, CA, USA



R. D. Arora (ed.), *Regenerative Medicine in Pain Practice*,
https://doi.org/10.1007/978-3-032-22644-0_12

**Barriers to Adoption**

- Lack of Public Awareness: Most potential patients do not understand what regenerative therapies are or how they work.
- Limited Physician Education: Referring doctors may lack exposure to or confidence in recommending regenerative options.
- Digital Confusion: Inconsistent, sometimes misleading online content creates skepticism.
- Regulatory Uncertainty: Evolving FDA (Food and Drug Administration) and FTC (Federal Trade Commission) guidelines can make clinicians hesitant to promote these services.
- Minimal Cross-Specialty Support: Orthopedics, rheumatology, and primary care may not yet embrace regenerative treatments.
- Lack of Standardization: Variability in procedures and outcomes diminishes confidence.
- Insufficient RCTs (Randomized Controlled Trials): The field lacks the volume of peer-reviewed studies that traditional medicine relies on.

## 12.3 The Author's Journey

My personal experience with regenerative therapies began not as a physician, but as a patient. After suffering knee and shoulder injuries, I underwent bone marrow cell therapy. The results were transformative, not only physically, but professionally. Motivated by this recovery, I pursued advanced training to learn more about the science behind regenerative medicine. This training afforded me expertise, which would allow me to offer regenerative therapy to my patients. I immersed myself in business and marketing strategies enabling me to integrate this therapy into my pain practice. My journey was filled with learning curves, experimentation, and growth. Through it all, I developed reproducible strategies that place patient education, transparency, and ethical practice at the forefront. I am sharing my story and exploits to illustrate how personal experience can lend authenticity and credibility to your practice.

## 12.4 Setting the Foundation: Important Marketing Principles

- Successful regenerative practices rest on a foundation of trust, education, and clear communication. The author, Dr. Arora, introduces three core pillars:
  - Evidence-Based Education: Patients are skeptical—provide them with real data and understandable explanations.
  - FDA Compliance: Avoid unproven claims. Stay within regulatory guidelines for all promotional activities.
  - Simple, Honest Messaging: Transparency builds credibility. Avoid hype; emphasize outcomes and safety. DO NOT over-sell.

I compare this to a preflight check. Just as a pilot thoroughly checks all systems before takeoff, a regenerative clinic must audit its messaging, branding, staff training, and legal compliance before launching marketing campaigns.

## 12.5 SWOT Analysis for Regenerative Clinics

A strategic SWOT analysis (Strengths, Weaknesses, Opportunities, Threats) helps clinics understand their internal and external environment:

| *Strengths* | *Weaknesses* |
|---|---|
| Physician credibility and reputation | New and unfamiliar to many patients |
| Innovative, non-surgical treatments | Confusing or contradictory online information |
| Freedom from insurance restrictions | Patients with negative past experiences |
| *Opportunities* | *Threats* |
| Market leadership in your region | Sudden changes in regulations |
| Direct patient communication | Encroachment by other specialties |
| Alternative revenue via cash services | Lack of hospital privileges or support |

## 12.6 Dr. Arora's 12 Steps to Regenerative Practice Success

*A roadmap for starting and scaling a regenerative medicine clinic:*

- Clarify your vision: Know why you're pursuing this field.
- Identify unmet needs: Where are current treatments falling short?
- Deepen your education: Attend hands-on and academic trainings.
- Learn marketing skills: Attend seminars focused on healthcare marketing.
- Develop a strategy: Tailor your marketing to your demographics and region.
- Build referral networks: Engage PCPs, PTs, chiropractors, and orthopedic colleagues.
- Brand yourself: Create a distinct identity for your regenerative services.
- Innovate: Stay ahead by incorporating evolving techniques.
- Set team goals: Align your staff with your mission.
- Comply with the FDA: Keep all patient-facing content within regulatory boundaries.
- Avoid hard selling: Inform, don't persuade. Educate patients to empower decisions.
- Focus on experience: Follow up, solicit feedback, and improve patient retention.

## 12.7 Multichannel Marketing Techniques

*An effective outreach strategy integrates traditional and digital platforms:*

- Patient-centric outreach.
- Community seminars and educational webinars.
- Magazine ads, direct mail, and flyers.
- Video testimonials and success stories.
- Clinic events and health fairs.
- Digital presence.
- Professional, optimized website with clear CTAs (Call To Action).
- SEO (Search Engine Optimization) and Google Ads targeting local search traffic.
- Educational social media posts (Instagram, Facebook, and YouTube).
- Patient-focused email newsletters.
- Online reputation management through reviews.

Consistency across all these channels ensures your message is clear, educational, and compliant.

## 12.8 Factors Patients Consider

Surveys indicate patients weigh several factors when choosing a provider:

- Physician credentials (73%): Patients trust board-certified, experienced clinicians.
- Cost (71%): Price transparency and financing options matter.
- Reviews and testimonials (57%): Positive feedback builds confidence.
- Payment plans (75%): Flexible options increase the likelihood of conversation.

Understanding these priorities helps tailor both your messaging and your service offerings.

## 12.9 Compliant Messaging: The Role of FDA and FTC

Regulatory bodies monitor the claims made about regenerative therapies:

FDA: Oversees the use and classification of biologics. Therapies involving minimally manipulated autologous cells must stay within 361 HCT/P criteria unless approved otherwise.

FTC: Ensures that marketing is truthful and not misleading.

*Tips for Compliance:*

- Avoid the term "stem cells" unless it accurately reflects FDA-recognized use.
- Focus on scientific mechanisms (e.g., "growth factors," "signal proteins").
- Share clinical outcomes backed by data, not promises of cure.
- Keep messaging balanced—highlight benefits while acknowledging limitations.

## 12.10 Enhancing Patient Loyalty

Loyalty is the byproduct of experience, empathy, and results. Practices that prioritize patient satisfaction see higher retention and word-of-mouth referrals.

*Loyalty Drivers:*

- Streamlined scheduling and minimal wait times.
- Compassionate, well-trained, and responsive staff.
- Clean, welcoming office environments.
- Proactive follow-ups and patient education.
- Open channels for questions and feedback.

Each patient encounter is an opportunity to build a long-term relationship.

## 12.11 Final Thoughts

The future of pain medicine is regenerative. But successful integration requires more than science, it requires vision, marketing acumen, and a commitment to ethical care.

*I emphasize, "Credibility is your most valuable currency."*

By combining regulatory compliance with patient-first messaging, regenerative practices can thrive in today's healthcare landscape. It is not about hype, it is about helping patients understand their options and giving them reasons to believe in your care.

## 12.12 Summary

Regenerative medicine offers clinicians a groundbreaking path forward in managing pain. However, success in this field depends not just on clinical skills but on strategic, patient-centered marketing. By embracing education, regulatory compliance, and principled communication, physicians can lead the way in this transformative era.

*Excuses will always be there for you—opportunity won't.*

*Good Luck in Regenerating the Practice!*
Ripu Arora 😊.

# Index




R. D. Arora (ed.), *Regenerative Medicine in Pain Practice*,
https://doi.org/10.1007/978-3-032-22644-0

MIX
Papier aus verantwortungsvollen Quellen
Paper from responsible sources
FSC® C105338

If you have any concerns about our products,
you can contact us on
**ProductSafety@springernature.com**

In case Publisher is established outside the EU,
the EU authorized representative is:
**Springer Nature Customer Service Center GmbH**
**Europaplatz 3, 69115 Heidelberg, Germany**

Printed by Libri Plureos GmbH
in Hamburg, Germany